The Myth of Alzheimer's

The Myth of Alzheimer's

WHAT YOU AREN'T BEING TOLD ABOUT TODAY'S MOST DREADED DIAGNOSIS

Peter J. Whitehouse, M.D., Ph.D.,
with
Daniel George, M.Sc.

St. Martin's Press ❧ New York

www.stmartins.com

Design by Maura Fadden Rosenthal/Mspace

Library of Congress Cataloging-in-Publication Data

Whitehouse, Peter J.
    The myth of Alzheimer's : what you aren't being told about today's most dreaded diagnosis / Peter J. Whitehouse with Daniel George. — 1st ed.
        p. cm.
        ISBN-13: 978-0-312-36816-6
        ISBN-10: 0-312-36816-X
    1. Alzheimer's disease—Popular works. I. George, Daniel (Daniel R.), 1982–
II. Title.
    RC523.2.W49 2007
    616.8'31—dc22   2007022176

First Edition: January 2008

10 9 8 7 6 5 4 3 2 1

CONTENTS

Authors' Note

In reflecting and writing on the emergence of Alzheimer's disease (AD) and its status in all of our lives, we have struggled to find the right tone with which to express our critique of the Alzheimer's field. Many of the professionals working in the field are Peter's friends. They are committed, hardworking people who have dedicated their lives to solving what is ostensibly one of our most dreaded "diseases."

Neither one of us wishes to cast aspersions, but we do wish to challenge the prevalently held assumptions in the Alzheimer's field—a field that seems to distort basic facts about brain aging and ignores the social implications of the monstrous Alzheimer's story it spreads; a field whose diagnostic categories have hardened and whose moral imagination has gradually dissipated; a field committed to treating the biology of a person's disease rather than focusing on the person who has the "disease" and the family who must adapt to the condition; a field that contributes to the separation of Alzheimer's "victims" from the rest of us while too often pursuing self-serving objectives.

By challenging the myth of AD, we wish to encourage our colleagues—especially those who deal with aging patients—to engage in a deep reflection about Alzheimer's disease, enable them to recognize the tremendous power that words and labels have in our lives, and consider the limits in our ability to cure a "disease" that we've built such a fearsome cultural myth around. The year 2007, the one hundredth anniversary of the publication of the first paper by Alois Alzheimer on the disease that now bears his name, presents such an opportunity for deep reflection.

We also want to reach out to individual readers who are coping with their own aging as well as the aging of loved ones. Peter's quarter-century in the field has convinced him that our entire approach to Alzheimer's disease needs to change. The unique stories that people and families bring to old age cannot be captured by the simplistic and reductionistic framework of Alzheimer's disease. Although Peter has applied (albeit reluctantly) the label of Alzheimer's disease to his patients for three decades, he now has come to realize the inadequacy of this label. Although he has participated in and even led the charge to find therapeutic approaches as a bench scientist, clinical trialist, and industry consultant, he now believes that there are better ways to approach improving the lives of those who seek his advice. We understand that *some* of the aging population seek the apparent comfort of a medical diagnosis and wish to honor these people, while proposing new ideas that can help reduce their suffering and bring about redemption during this great personal and familial struggle. Peter's hope is that the ideas and values expressed in this book can help his current and future patients enjoy a better quality of life as they age.

The baby boomer generation is going to revolutionize the way we age, and will continue to challenge the conventions of retirement and old age that held true for their parents. They have been creative risk takers and will continue to aspire to the highest quality of life as they age. Their wisdom, knowledge, and resources will potentially transform our cultural approach to retirement, while their sense of purpose (and perhaps entitlement) will do away with many of the stereotypes, stigmas, and prejudices we have about old age. We are entering a complicated era as a human species in which new health priorities are emerging, and new ways of thinking about our aging society and our aging bodies and minds are much needed.

To bring about a new framework that can help us adapt to aging in the twenty-first century, Alzheimer's disease has to be talked about, brought out into the open, and seen from a more enlightened perspective. If we engage in a genuine and open dialogue with the myth of Alzheimer's disease, we will all learn a great deal about ourselves. Most important, we can begin to be emancipated from conventional and outmoded approaches to brain aging. After all, there is no single way to describe aging. By challenging the framework of Alzheimer's disease—a framework that is not especially salient or helpful to the lives of emerging elders and is severely limited in its scope—we can begin to envision new strategies for successful aging in the twenty-first century.

For those of us who want to reframe the way our culture views aging and venture forth in telling our own story about growing older at this critical juncture in human history, we welcome your participation in ending Alzheimer's and bringing about a better and more genuinely hopeful and healthy future for aging human beings—and hence for all of us.

PREFACE

*T*he Myth of Alzheimer's will give you a new perspective on brain aging that will help you and your family members better understand Alzheimer's disease (AD)—what Alzheimer's is and isn't, who stands to gain from your being labeled with Alzheimer's, and, most important, how you can steer clear of the AD diagnosis, maintain the quality of your brain and the quality of your life as you age, and derive meaning rather than dread from the aging process. You will also learn how our society can help families and communities adapt to the challenges of brain aging and what we as individuals can do to move the process forward.

I don't have a magic bullet to prevent brain aging, and I don't claim to have the cure for AD, but I do offer a powerful therapy—a new story for approaching brain aging that undercuts the destructive Alzheimer's myth we tell today. As my friend and colleague Mark Turner has written, narrative imagination—the ability to tell stories—is the fundamental instrument of our thought. Most of our knowledge and our thinking is organized in story form, and thus stories offer us the chief means of making sense of the present, looking into the future, and planning and creating our lives.[1] Developing a new approach to brain aging requires a new story that can move us beyond the myth of Alzheimer's disease and toward improved quality of life for all aging persons in our society.

SETTING THE SCENE

Today in the United States, the average life span is in the low eighties for women and the mid-seventies for men. As you move along the path to old age, you should be able to do so on your own terms and not be unduly influenced or guided by a medical profession and drug industry that may not always have your best interests at heart. The landscape of aging is changing in the twenty-first century, and the simplistic, uni-dimensional view of Alzheimer's disease is beginning to crumble.

In other countries, life expectancy is greater than the United States, despite our disproportionate wealth. As a society, we need to ask why this is so.

This book will challenge the conventional wisdom and assumptions about AD. It will enlighten you, give you hope about your own aging, urge you to throw away the stigmatizing labels that doctors like me have been too quick to apply, and help you move forward on your journey toward older age. If nothing else, it will better inform you by telling the fascinating story of how a single "peculiar" medical case observed by Dr. Alois Alzheimer in 1906 became known as a full-blown disease that has grown into a $100-billion-a-year marketing and research juggernaut, with more than 25 million people afflicted worldwide.[2]

In this book I will answer these questions:

- Is Alzheimer's even a disease?

- What is the difference between a naturally aging brain and an Alzheimer's brain?

- How effective are the current drugs for AD? Are they worth the money we spend on them?

- What kind of hope does science really have for the treatment of memory loss? Are there alternative interventions that can keep our aging bodies and minds sharp?

- What promise does genetic research actually hold?

- What would a world without Alzheimer's look like, and how do we as individuals and as human communities get there?

Part One and Part Two will expose the unsound clinical, political, and scientific framework of Alzheimer's disease and explain why it continues to be so difficult to treat or cure the condition.

Part Three explores preventive measures that can be taken to reduce the risk for cognitive aging, and presents examples of how to maintain cognitive vitality and a sense of fulfillment and social contribution as we age. I will provide practical answers for when it's time to see a doctor for memory loss and explain how to find the right medical team, how to establish your voice in the clinic, and how to develop a collaborative relationship with your physician as you face the challenges of brain aging. Because I have worked with thousands of patients with varying levels of cognitive challenges, I also offer advice on how you and your family can integrate memory loss into your lives and face the worst-case scenario: a diagnosis of AD. Having this enriched perspective—this new story built on a solid foundation of knowledge—will help you make decisions for yourself and for your loved ones, reduce your stress, and give you the hope, purpose, and guidance to age gracefully and meaningfully as you embark on the challenging journey of brain aging.

OVERCOMING THE TYRANNY OF AD

This book does not diminish the very real needs of those who suffer from the deepest throes of senility, impaired bodily functions, wandering, mood changes, delusions and hallucinations, and dependence on twenty-four-hour care. I'm speaking out against the traditional view of AD that has been ingrained in all of us—that those afflicted with a "disease" called Alzheimer's suffer a total and devastating loss of self resulting from a pathological event while the rest of us cower in fear of our own aging and wait for a biological cure. Neurodegenerative conditions do not "claim" older people, nor do they dominate them or degrade their humanity; they simply alter the manner by which we live our lives. *As you will learn in this book, there is no such thing as an "Alzheimer's victim," no such thing as a total "loss of self." The disease is never bigger than the person.*

The myth of Alzheimer's would have us think differently. Many of those first diagnosed with Alzheimer's, or its so-called precursor, Mild Cognitive Impairment (MCI), worry that their decline may be a fast free fall into total memory loss—a veritable "loss of self," an "erosion of selfhood," "a never-ending funeral."

AN IMPORTANT RULE OF THUMB

As a physician who has been privileged to work closely with many patients over the last three decades, I can tell you that everyone's brain ages along a different trajectory. Some brains age along a gentle curve; others slope downward more rapidly; still others curve slowly and then dip at the end. When seeing patients, I will sometimes hold out my left hand parallel to the floor to illustrate this point, explaining that the trajectory along which people age varies in the same way my five fingers aim. My thumb can actually point up—some people improve—but my spread fingers show varying rates of decline. Although we will all gradually lose some of our cognitive abilities as we age, *The Myth of Alzheimer's* will show readers there is no such thing as "Alzheimer's disease" that *claims* elderly victims or erodes our personhood—no one trajectory or series of progressive

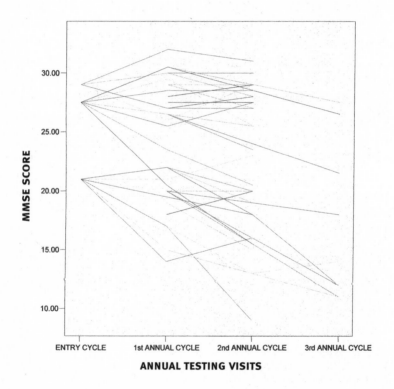

Figure 1. The Variability of Brain Aging.   Each line represents a single participant in our research program over time (up to three years). Data from other centers around the world would look the same. The Mini Mental State Examination (MMSE) is a simple test of cognitive abilities with scores ranging from 0 to 30 (best). The graph shows three groups of people tested several times: normal persons (top line with best scores all arbitrarily "normalized" to be starting from the same point), persons diagnosed with Mild Cognitive Impairment, and persons diagnosed with Alzheimer's disease (lowest starting scores). The rates of change over time are quite variable, with much overlap among the three groups. In fact, in some cases, persons with dementia will improve on their scores—there is no one trajectory of decline for Alzheimer's disease, MCI, or normal aging. (Data analysis and display courtesy of McKee McClendon, University Memory and Aging Center, University Hospitals Case Medical Center)

stages[3] that we are all fated to advance along should we be given the AD or MCI label.

This is not merely a semantics issue over *Alzheimer's* versus *senility*. Scientists still can't agree upon what Alzheimer's is. As you will see, it is a disease without a clear-cut definition; there is no agreed-upon way to differentiate AD from normal aging, making every diagnosis only "possible" or "probable," and every individual case heterogeneous and unique in its course. Existing treatments are not effective, and talk of "a cure" is based on faith, not measured scientific extrapolations. One thing we do know is that Alzheimer's is a multibillion-dollar industry, and that the label is driven in large part by the pharmaceutical industry and by some academic experts and others who use the exaggerated characterization of AD entrepreneurially to promote maximum concern for dementia and therefore maximize research support of the disorder and sustain the clinical empire that has been built around it. The medical story of AD generates fear, paranoia, angst, and stigmatization while evoking powerful social and emotional images. A diagnosis of AD can act in many ways as a death sentence of the mind, which imprisons many still-functional adults to a mental death row. By trying to de-stigmatize cognitive decline with a disease label that takes the onus off the person, we have actually made the ostracism of the sufferers worse. The words we use to describe diseases have the potential to do emotional and social harm.

> Remember that diseases can come and go. When speaking, I often tell audiences that, in the 1800s, "drapetomania" was considered a disease that caused slaves to run away! In our present day, aging is being considered by some as a disease to be cured.[4]

This current framework—this *myth* of Alzheimer's—prevents us from seeing the potential for vitality, fulfillment, and even wisdom that still exists along the slope of our declining years. In *The Myth of Alzheimer's,* I will take on the powerful forces that have shaped these erroneous and misleading views, and liberate our minds and bodies from the tyranny of the Alzheimer's disease story so that we may choose to walk the path of aging on our own terms.

> *To conquer fear is the beginning of wisdom.*
> —BERTRAND RUSSELL

Creating a new framework for brain aging can change not only our beliefs and attitudes about aging, but it can also change our options for healing as we grow older. Thinking about brain aging not as a disease, but as a lifelong process fraught with challenges, will change our whole approach to aging and add quality to our later years and to the lives of those we love. In fact, at the heart of a more enlightened view of Alzheimer's is a more optimistic and realistic view of what it means to be an aging human being in relationship to others who are growing older. The language we use matters a great deal. If we can learn to think and speak about brain aging differently—to tell a different story about ourselves as we age—we can better assist individuals and families in coping with cognitive decline.

MY PERSPECTIVE

For the last thirty years, I have worked as a geriatric neurologist and seen thousands of patients struggling with the challenges of brain aging. In the 1980s, discoveries that I made as a researcher at Johns Hopkins University contributed to the development of the first drugs approved to treat AD. Although I continue to speak about what I used to call "Alzheimer's disease" at conferences around the world, and, until 2007, consulted on drug development with the pharmaceutical industry, I have slowly adapted my practice and moved away from the mainstream biomedical approach in order to provide better care for patients. Some may consider my approach unorthodox but I have often been voted one of the Top Doctors in America, and my patients regularly commend me for the nature of care they receive.

A LETTER FROM A PATIENT

"My husband has been a patient of Dr. Whitehouse since first showing early signs of dementia about ten years ago. I doubt that my husband or I would be as emotionally sound or as functional today without Dr. Whitehouse's caring and capable support. Both from his knowledge of (in some cases cutting-edge) medications to his attentive monitoring of my husband's capabilities, Dr. Whitehouse has been a godsend to my husband. And, perhaps even more important, the guidance and emotional reinforcement Dr. Whitehouse has provided me as my husband's caregiver has encouraged me and propped me up during this difficult challenge. His loving, empathetic, personal medical style is a throwback to the country doctors of a century ago."

—Helen Kranz, Spring 2006

Outside of the clinic, I have consulted for many multinational drug companies, including serving on numerous advisory boards, receiving on average $50,000 to $75,000 of additional income each year for the past twenty years—well over a total of a million dollars in personal income over the course of my career. I have also received grants to support various research and educational activities totaling several million more. As the developer of the International Working Group for the Harmonization of Dementia Drug Guidelines (a group focused on improving the efficiency of drug development) and a leader in numerous international organizations, I have traveled the world helping to develop more effective interventions for AD and related disorders. Many of these trips were subsidized by drug industry dollars.

My engagement with industry has enabled me to understand pharmaceutical companies from a revealing insider perspective and discover the sources of strength as well as some of the mechanisms of deception they deploy. My efforts have earned me a modicum of influence with drug companies, and the right to present my vision for how they and the medical field should act as agents for world benefit rather than stockholder benefit. I am well aware of the social forces at work in the Alzheimer's field as a result of my years of experience, and now I want to share what I've learned with as broad a readership as possible, including those associated with the pharmaceutical industry and Alzheimer's organizations.

While *The Myth of Alzheimer's* aims to change the way pharmaceutical companies do business, it is at root a book for aging baby boomers, health-care professionals, and anyone else who wants to join me in bringing a new understanding to Alzheimer's disease and taking control of their own brain aging.

> *Every human being is the author of his own health or disease.*
>
> —THE BUDDHA

THE HISTORY OF A DISEASE

REVEALING THE MYTH OF ALZHEIMER'S

If at first the idea is not absurd,
then there is no hope.

—ALBERT EINSTEIN

When we think about myths, we usually think of timeless tales of gods, heroes, and monsters that entertain and enthrall. Since the Enlightenment, mythology has been regarded as the province of more primitive minds—something humanity has moved beyond in its embrace of scientific methodology. But *has* science been successful in purging contemporary civilization of all myths? I don't believe that it has or likely ever will.

In fact, although we depend on the objectivity of science, scientifically influenced fields such as medicine are often rife with their own myths and misapprehensions. This is because, as the anthropologist Claude Lévi-Strauss[1] believed, every myth—whether it be about a god hurling a lightning bolt from a mountain, a hero undertaking harrowing adventures filled with sirens, storms, and ferocious beasts, or a generation of scientists trying to fight a peculiar disease of old age—is driven by the need to address the complexities of the human condition and to try to resolve paradoxes that perplex us. In our modern age, in which remarkable scientific and technological advances have both extended and brought quality to human lives, we find major challenges to our rationality and values as science attempts to understand our own mysterious organ of rational thought—the brain—and the very processes of brain aging. From out of the depths of this paradox, a hundred-year-old monster has risen; it is called "Alzheimer's disease."

THE MYTH OF ALZHEIMER'S

Alzheimer's disease represents our culture's attempt to make sense of a natural process (brain aging) that we cannot control. Just as past civilizations posited mythical explanations for natural events they could not explain, we have created an antagonist: a terrorizing disease of the brain that our scientists are fighting against. The pillars of the myth are as follows:

AD is a singular disease

Despite widespread belief that there is a disease called Alzheimer's against which science is waging war, what the public isn't told is that so-called Alzheimer's disease cannot be differentiated from normal aging and that no two illness courses are the same. As you will learn, there is no one biological profile of Alzheimer's that is consistent from person to person, and all the biological hallmarks of AD are also the hallmarks of normal brain aging.

People "get" Alzheimer's in old age

It seems as if more people fall victim to Alzheimer's each year. Newspapers and magazines would have us believe that Alzheimer's is spreading throughout human populations, and especially baby boomers, like an epidemic and claiming millions more victims.

However, what you aren't told is that we don't even know how to diagnose Alzheimer's disease, let alone tabulate the numbers of disease victims. Because there is no single biological profile for AD, every clinical diagnosis is considered "probable"—and, frankly speaking, not even postmortem examination can differentiate a so-called AD victim from those who have aged normally. Hence, the claim that a diagnosis of "definite" Alzheimer's can be made after death is itself questionable. The gold standard of neuropathology is a bit tarnished. No one really ever "gets" a singular disease called Alzheimer's, and there is no evidence that Alzheimer's is spreading throughout the baby boomer population other than the fact that the world is aging and there are more middle-aged people at risk for brain-aging phenomena.

We can cure Alzheimer's through the continued investment of our public and private dollars

The myth that Alzheimer's is a disease separate from aging also carries the promise that science will one day win the "war" against this disease. But if Alzheimer's cannot be differentiated from normal brain aging, to cure AD we would literally have to arrest the natural process of brain aging. I am not alone in casting doubt upon this myth. As you will read, even scientists in the Alzheimer's research field will tell you that a cure is unlikely and that we need to invest our dollars more wisely by putting them toward prevention and care rather than predominantly in cure. However, like the myth of the Fountain of Youth, which captivated past civilizations, the promise of a panacea for one of our most dreaded "diseases" is a powerful cultural myth, and one purveyed by powerful pharmaceutical companies, advocacy organizations, and private researchers with much profit to gain. It is a myth we have been seduced by, and the combination of hype and fear it inspires has distorted our expectations and understandings about our aging brains.

MY STORY

For nearly twenty-five years, I have served as a leader in the Alzheimer's field, and have helped international Alzheimer's organizations and pharmaceutical companies shape the rules, guidelines, diagnostic categories, and accepted clinical approaches to Alzheimer's disease. My experiences and relationships with other colleagues have endowed me with some influence and power and have enabled me to become what the science community calls a "thought leader" (or KOL—"key opinion leader")—one who guides our conventional thinking about a particular condition.

In the beginning of my career, at a time when no medicines had been approved specifically for Alzheimer's and companies were unsure about how to proceed in drug development, the pharmaceutical industry reached out to me and listened to my thoughts and opinions about treating persons with memory challenges. Once drugs made their way to the market in the 1990s the relationship shifted. Rather than being interested in having my thoughts influence their views, it seemed as if industry wanted to change *my* mind and convince me that their drugs were worth giving to my patients. This focus on biological approaches to brain aging across our society has shifted the whole dynamic of the field away from caring for the aging patient and his family and toward drugs as the primary means of ensuring the quality of his life. Too often, aging patients and their families leave the doctor's office with little more than a pill prescription (often encompassing several pills) and fear generated by the Alzheimer's myth, knowing little about how to effectively care for the condition.

This is inhumane and inexcusable.

Now, upon the one hundredth anniversary of the first case of Alzheimer's, I feel obliged to share my stories and the insight I have gained, to inform the general public how I—a lifelong Alzheimer's disease researcher and clinician—have evolved to espouse a different ideological position that transforms a significant portion of what I've believed in as a professional carer for patients. Having spent my life within the scientific, political, economic, and social institutions of the AD field—universities, hospitals, pharmaceutical companies—studying and treating human aging and disease, I am ready to challenge the power that the mainstream "Alzheimer's disease" myth has over us and help people see what I have seen and to think critically about the evolution in thought that has occurred over the past several decades, which has shaped the way we see our aging bodies and minds and the way we act toward them. I want to articulate a story of brain aging that can be a starting point for helping us better cope with and prepare for the travails of cognitive decline.

No longer can we safely assume that the march of progress in the "War against AD" is moving at the hoped for speed or direction; no longer can we maintain the mythical illusion that AD is a battle against a specific disease that we will eventually "win"; no longer can we keep looking at aging persons, however embattled, as somehow "diseased." *Defining brain aging as a disease and then trying to cure it is at its root unscientific and misguided. In short, Alzheimer's is a hundred-year old myth that is over the hill. The entire scientific, technological, and political framework for aging needs to be reassessed to better serve patients and families in order to help people maximize their quality of life as they move along the path of cognitive aging.*

THE STORY OF FRANK AND FRAN

Frank J.

68 years old

6'2"

186 lbs.

Concerned about short-term memory lapses

Frank is a retired newspaper editor from Boston, whose short-term memory lapses have him frightened that he has Alzheimer's. Fearing the worst, he has explored the Alzheimer's Association Web site to learn more about his condition. "Alzheimer's disease," the Web site says, "is a progressive brain disorder that gradually destroys a person's memory and ability to learn, reason, make judgments, communicate and carry out daily activities." Frank gets the name of a local neurologist from one of his doctor friends and intends to set up an appointment.

Fran W.

57 years old

5'6"

135 lbs.

Memory problems and spatial disorientation

Fran is a retired children's librarian who has been experiencing memory problems that have thrown her world into disorder. She frequently forgets the time and date and has become anxious, and even obsessive, about her bills and mail, which she's been stowing in shoeboxes underneath her bed in an elaborately organized system. Three weeks ago, she became disoriented behind the wheel and drove into a nearby Baltimore suburb, where she was given a ticket for nearly causing an accident by turning left from the right-hand lane. Fran's family has been worried about her, especially because her father died twenty-five years ago with severe dementia. Her family has convinced her to make an appointment with a neurologist recommended by a friend.

Fran and Frank both visit their doctors with family members—Frank with his son Patrick, and Fran with her daughter Beth.

Frank's doctor enters the room in a harried manner and offers quick handshakes to him and Patrick. Opening up Frank's chart, he asks Frank to describe his memory problems and then conducts a physical examination. They cycle through hearing, vision, and strength-and-sensation tests, and the doctor silently jots notes in his chart. He then gives Frank a brief memory test, during which Frank curses out loud because it's clear that the fog is in his head today.

"You know, Doctor, I was a journalist, and I'm used to boiling a story down to the basic facts," Frank says. "I may not like what I hear, but when you tell me what I have, I want you to tell it to me straight. If it's Alzheimer's, tell me it's Alzheimer's."

The doctor nods and tells him, "It may in fact be a case of Alzheimer's. I'm not going to make that diagnosis until we get the results of your tests back."

He arranges several procedures for Frank—a lumbar puncture to measure amyloid and tau proteins in the cerebrospinal fluid (CSF), along with two brain scans (an MRI and PET) and a neuropsychological examination. He also orders a blood test to find out whether Frank has the ApoE-4 gene. Frank tries to maintain his composure, but the prospect of undergoing multiple tests and the fear about what they might show make him feel nauseated and scared.

On the return appointment two weeks later, the neurologist enters the exam room carrying Frank's patient record and the results of his tests. After a quick exchange of pleasantries, he gets right to the point:

"Your neurological exam showed the patterns of problems with naming and memory that we associate with Alzheimer's. In addition, your brain imaging and CSF tests are consistent with this diagnosis, and we have identified that you are a carrier of the ApoE-4 gene. This puts you at a higher risk for developing Alzheimer's disease than the normal person. So, in short, Frank, I can tell you that you have Alzheimer's disease."

Frank shifts uncomfortably in his chair, a fog of nausea merging with the fog of his confusion. There is a brief pause, and then the doctor continues, directing his attention to Patrick.

"It's not the end of the world. We have safe and effective drugs called cholinesterase inhibitors, which I'll put your father on right away. I presume that's okay with you?"

Frank looks down at his hands, and then glances at Patrick, who fixes his gaze at the floor and nods his consent.

"Well, Doctor," says Frank hoarsely, gathering himself. "I can't say this comes as a shock, but it's certainly hard news to take. I just don't want to be a burden." He pauses. "Doctor . . . can you tell me I'm not just going to fade away like my mother did? Can you tell me I'm not going to just lose myself to Alzheimer's?"

Fran's visit starts more auspiciously than Frank's. She and her daughter Beth meet the doctor and are pleased to find that he's a personable man. All of them strike a quick rapport. The doctor listens as Fran talks about her days as a librarian, her hobbies, her family—about when she last felt herself to be sound of mind. Though Fran is having trouble speaking today, mostly because of nerves, the doctor encourages her to tell the story of her memory problems and how they've affected her daily life and her relationships with the rest of her family.

Without speaking, she pulls out her purse and passes the doctor a small framed photograph.

It's a picture of her father dressed in his Navy uniform.

"My dad had dementia. He died twenty-five years ago. Watching him fade away was . . . just . . . just . . . well, worse than you could ever imagine. But now my mind is dimming just like his did. I'm so afraid I'm going to be a burden on my family," she tells him.

The doctor nods reassuringly. He asks Fran whether she has consulted with anyone outside the medical community about her condition, or sought help from a complementary and alternative medicine provider, or talked with someone in the religious community. He encourages Fran to maintain hope rather than fear.

The doctor proceeds to tell Fran that she will be given a neuropsychological test, which will measure her intellectual strengths and her creativity in addition to her weaknesses. Otherwise, she will not be subjected to any invasive tests, which comes as a great relief to Fran. They will meet again in a week's time to follow up.

The next week, the doctor invites Fran and Beth to accompany him to his office. He asks how Fran is doing and listens as she talks about the reading she has been doing. Recently, she has returned her books on Alzheimer's and borrowed two self-help books on successful aging: *The Creative Age* by Gene Cohen, and *Finding Meaning in the Second Half of Life* by James Hollis.

"Well, Fran," he tells her, "I think this is an opportune time to review the results of your test, which were actually quite positive. What they showed me was that though your visual-spatial capacity may be relatively weak, you are still very strong in verbal performance, which I would fully expect from someone who has spent her life around books."

Fran nods, and then looks the doctor in the eye.

"But you need to tell me, Doctor: Do I have a disease? Do I have Alzheimer's like my dad?"

"Well, Fran, you have what other people might label as 'Alzheimer's disease,' but I don't believe that type of label applies well to your situation. All people have brains that age over time, and all of our brains age in different ways. Some people lose some spatial abilities and some lose verbal abilities—no two cases of brain aging are ever the same. There is remarkable variability in the clinical course of what people used to call Alzheimer's disease. The trajectory of every aging person is unique.

"It's important that you know that you're not alone in your memory problems and that you're not diseased, even though your memory loss may be more pronounced than others your age. Almost everybody gets memory problems to one degree or another as they grow older—unfortunately, some people are more affected than others."

"But will I end up like my dad?"

"I am afraid no one can predict your pattern of change over time. But you are not going to fade away, it's never that simple," the doctor says.

"This does not have to be a tragedy," he goes on. "Even though you're aging, you are still a vital human being with cognitive strengths who can contribute to your family and to society and explore your creative potential. Think of your brain as an old book. Even though it may be a bit tattered, a little worn around the edges, it still possesses wisdom, knowledge, and value that can be given to others."

"Thank you, Doctor," Beth says. "But I still would like to know what my mom has."

The doctor nods. "Beth, after all my years as a neurologist, I have become convinced that we need to break free from the mind-set that memory loss is some sort of a 'disease' that someone 'gets.' Your mom's memory loss is part of what my colleagues and I are coming to understand as the variable results of brain aging. Though it may sound a bit strange, Alzheimer's disease cannot be diagnosed—it's a construct that science doesn't fully understand, which I don't believe is very helpful in situations like yours. There is a better framework we can use to explain your mom's condition."

The doctor turns to Fran.

"I think that it's better to think of this as a challenging condition that puts you and your family in difficult circumstances you must adapt to. Now, obviously, the next logical question to ask is, What can you do? This is the most important part of successful aging."

The doctor spends the next ten minutes talking to her about making dietary changes, eating more fruits and vegetables, as well as foods high in antioxidants, B vitamins, and fish, which is high in omega-3 fatty acids that also seem to have cardio-protective benefits in addition to cognitive ones. He explains the importance of diet in keeping cholesterol and blood pressure low and reducing the risk for diabetes.

"But what's even more important than what you eat is with whom you eat," he says.

With that, he urges her to stay socially and physically active and recommends walking outdoors in warm weather and then in indoor malls when it gets cold; he also emphasizes the importance of continuing to play bridge with friends and meeting them for dinner every week. He suggests taking classes through the adult education program in the community building on the other side of town where she can paint, write, put together an ethical will, play cards, learn calming meditation techniques—"anything that will keep you active and engaged," as he puts it.

Lastly, he tells Fran that there are drugs available for her condition, which could offer some small benefit and may be worth a try. He stresses that it is more important that she focus on other ways of staying cognitively vital and to adjust emotionally to the reality of her changing memory, and says that Fran's health team at the clinic—a nurse and social worker—will help her do this.

"Remember," he tells Fran. "Your life has purpose, and part of that purpose is to continue to help others, just as you have done in the past with your family and with your work in libraries."

Beth reaches over to hold her mother's hand as the doctor continues.

"Fran, I'd also like to suggest that with your verbal strengths, and your experience as a librarian, you enroll in a research project I have started, in which you will teach young kids from the inner city to read. This is an intergenerational initiative that will help people like you find purpose in their later years while allowing you to contribute your skills to a community that really needs them."

Fran laughs. "I'm a librarian, Doctor—we're not allowed to like kids!" Nevertheless, she agrees to give the volunteering a try.

The doctor thanks Fran and Beth for coming, and on the way out says, "The most important thing is that I don't want you living in fear of

Alzheimer's disease, Fran. You are still a vital person who can find purpose and fulfillment in your life and contribute to your family and to your community, even with your aging brain. Your family and I are going to work together to help you write a story of successful aging."

THE WISDOM OF FRANK AND FRAN

In these stories, Frank and Fran have exhibited clinical symptoms that would qualify them for the Alzheimer's disease label, but each received a different clinical story from their doctor that drastically altered the outlook of their condition. Frank's doctor orders a battery of invasive tests, which all seem to indicate that his patient has the deficits of Alzheimer's. In consequence, Frank is given a probable AD diagnosis—the standard story—and is immediately put on cholinesterase inhibitor pills to treat the condition. Understanding himself to be an "Alzheimer's" victim, Frank fears that the disease will doom him to a slow, passive demise and render him a burden on his son. Frank's doctor feels that he has given him a basic biomedical framework in which to understand his cognitive degeneration and draw hope. In reality, this corrupted cultural myth of AD places Frank at the center of a fearsome story with a tragic trajectory that plunges him into suffering and woe.

On the other hand, Fran exemplifies how a patient with memory challenges can be uplifted by her interaction with a physician—how a more humane and empathetic story about the brain-aging process can combine clinical reality with personal narrative and a vision of hope that can empower elderly persons to realize their human potential and age successfully even as they lose some of their cognitive abilities. Fran's doctor has realized the harm caused by the dominant story of Alzheimer's disease and is actively assisting his patients in creating their own story in place of the standard AD myth. Unlike Frank, who received a disease label, a prescription for cholinesterase inhibitors, and a promise that more effective treatments were on the horizon—as happens to hundreds of thousands of people each year—Fran received a comprehensive strategy of bio-psychosocial care that would allow her to maintain independent functioning and feel a sense of normality, connectedness, and social and familial usefulness despite her cognitive challenges.

Fran's memory problems and her persistent worries about becoming her father were not denied, ignored, or trivialized by her neurologist. Instead, the doctor allayed her anxiety about Alzheimer's disease by telling a different story about cognitive aging—a scientifically honest one that de-emphasized the disease label and offered a plan of action to Fran rather than contributing to her fears. While Frank frets about being stigmatized by the label and fatalistically resigns himself to fading away, Fran understands that experiencing memory challenges places her in a majority rather than a minority. The doctor is fostering a story that will enable Fran to age with dignity on her own terms instead of dying disgraced within an intimidating disease framework.

Now I'm going to tell you a small secret: The doctor who treated Frank also provided care for Fran. And in both cases I was that doctor.

I have met thousands of patients like Frank and Fran. Frank is a modern composite of the patients who came to me when I was a young physician at Johns Hopkins University in the 1980s, an endlessly rational, technology-oriented professional who saw what I then called Alzheimer's disease as a pathological disease that could be cured with neurotherapeutics. I emphasized the tragedy in cognitive aging and the burden of caregiving rather than the hope that still remained for affected persons and the potential for growth for their family. Fran is a composite patient who saw the doctor I have become: a committed healer for my elderly patients.

Frank and Fran can have real implications for how our society cares for our aging men and women in the twenty-first century. I am enacting Fran's story with other patients in my own clinical practice and encouraging my colleagues to do so as well. Every aspect of Fran's successful aging plan is real. My patients in Cleveland are:

- Eating healthier diets

- Staying physically fit

- Participating in book clubs

- Volunteering in various programs with inner-city children who are learning to read, utilizing local resources to learn new skills, staying cognitively vital, and keeping socially engaged

- Participating in structured conversations designed to guide families through difficult decision making at the end of life

In other words, my patients and I have begun imagining a new story of brain aging that triumphs over the myth of Alzheimer's. I am finding that a more scientifically honest and humanistic framework of brain aging will enhance the quality of life of those with cognitive challenges who find themselves under medical supervision and care, as well as their families. Clinically, I have ceased promoting the AD diagnosis to describe the cognitive aging process in my patients and have de-emphasized the use of cholinesterase inhibitors to treat the symptoms of brain aging. I am more attentive to my patients' stories, and integrate their memory problems into an ongoing narrative that they themselves help write rather than ushering them into the terrifying and nonredemptive myth that medicine has written for them.

THE ROLE OF SCIENCE IN THE NEW STORY OF BRAIN AGING

I have not abandoned my belief in science, nor my hope that we will one day find better ways to protect the brain against the effects of aging. As the Dalai Lama says, we human beings must constantly devote ourselves to seeking new knowledge. It's part of our nature. However, I believe the myth of Alzheimer's is causing us to waste massive resources in unwise quests for magic bullets to "fix" brain aging—putting cure before care and prevention, and trying to achieve dominance over a domain that will continue to resist our control. Biotechnology infatuates our collective imaginations, and deserves a reasonable investment of our resources—but more profound answers lie in us as individuals and members of caring communities than in the databases and therapy models proposed by scientists, who are working

---

DEMENTIA RECONSIDERED

"One of the consequences of depathologizing dementia is that there is no supreme medical authority to whom one might look for definitive answers, and there are no technical solutions, ready-made, on which to rely. . . . In one sense this is cause for relief; there is no need to continue [the] vigil in the temple of biomedical science that we have had to endure so long. In another sense, however, it presents an enormous challenge, because it means a full acceptance of responsibility; we must find all the main resources for caring within ourselves."[2]

—Tom Kitwood, British psychologist, 1937–1998

with incomplete theories about how the brain works and how memory loss comes about.

The infatuation with technology makes us forget to do such simple preventive things to protect our brains from cognitive loss as wearing a bicycle helmet, eating healthy, exercising, or ensuring pure public drinking water without toxins like lead, arsenic, methylmercury, and PCBs, which damage brain tissue, or providing all children with access to the nutrients that the brain needs to grow and develop. It also persuades our lawmakers to invest disproportionately in the search for the cure, when really our resources would be much better off invested in building communities that can help families care for the large number of aging persons in the twenty-first century.

WRITING THE NEW STORY OF BRAIN AGING

As the British author Philip Pullman says, stories may not be the best medicine, but they are nutritious and sustaining.[3] They feed the mind with information and the heart with hope and strength. Nature and medical science together can do a great deal to help our bodies and minds heal themselves, but having a better story in which to frame our inevitable mental and physical aging can give us the nourishment that sustains us as we grow older.

> **QUOTE TO PONDER**
>
> "A good story, perhaps, is essential to a sense of self-worth"
>
> —Robert Fulford, journalist

And so, what it comes down to is this: Would you rather be part of Frank's story or Fran's? Would you prefer a traditional clinical encounter like Frank's in which you are given a terminal disease label, told that a cure does not exist, and routed into the "find a cure" track of biological research? Or would you rather be in Fran's position: having your suffering recognized and honored without bearing the albatross of an Alzheimer's label; being offered an opportunity to participate in a community service research study in which you would contribute to your community and to subsequent generations of kids?

Which story would you rather tell for yourself?

The charge of this book is to move us past the current myth of Alzheimer's—the story that shapes the reality of so many who are aging—and the best time to start is now. So where does the change begin? It starts with you. As William James once wrote, human beings, by changing the inner attitudes of their minds, can change the outer aspects of their lives. Language is the tool we can use to activate a new story for brain aging. To think differently, we must speak differently.

> QUOTE TO PONDER
>
> **"If we spoke a different language, we would perceive a somewhat different world."**
>
> —Ludwig Wittgenstein

What follows are small, subtle, but important modifications we can make in our everyday speech and thought that can help us rise above the terror, fear, and despairing metaphors of the Alzheimer's myth and manifest a better future for ourselves. I expect that many of these modifications will look peculiar upon first glance. But when you are finished with *The Myth of Alzheimer's,* I hope you can return to them with your enriched perspective, and that this new language of brain aging can begin to enter into your self-understanding and into the conversations you have with others.

AD is a brain disease →Brain aging is variable

We will learn that Alzheimer's is not a specific brain disease. It can not be diagnosed definitively in life or death nor does it have one basic defining pathological feature. *Alzheimer's disease* as a term for brain aging is a misnomer that militarizes our understanding of our bodies, causes us to denigrate and exclude those with the "disease," and also does grave injustice to Dr. Alois Alzheimer, who, despite never really believing that the condition he observed in his first patient, Auguste D., should be distinguished as a separate disease entity, now has his name attached to one of humanity's most dreaded ailments.

A humanistic, ecological framework of *brain aging* acknowledges the hardships and challenges of old age, while enabling us to avoid the stigma of a mental illness label. Instead of using "mythical" language and talking about a "mind-wasting" disease that "steals the selfhood" of our loved ones, and fighting a valiant "war against Alzheimer's" in search of a biological fix, we can use words like *personhood, integrity,* and *dignity* to refer to those who are aging, and words like *balance, quality of life, responsibility for future generations, community, prevention,* and *conservation* to reframe our individual and cultural priorities.[4] Such language can lead us away from the notion that the individual brain (or genome) is a site of a war that can be won, and toward a consideration of population health that respects the frailty and limits of human life and places a greater emphasis on preventing and caring for cognitive loss rather than "fixing" it. By thinking about Alzheimer's as a molecular disease at the end of life, we are only seeing the puddles of cognitive aging and ignoring the rainstorm that occurs throughout life. We must look at brain aging holistically, as a process that occurs from womb to tomb, so that we can see from the vantage of youth the gathering clouds of cognitive decline and protect ourselves from the hard rain that falls on all of us as we age.

AD ravages the brain → Brain aging creates age-associated cognitive challenges

Our militarized understanding of AD causes us to see brain aging as a singular disease that ravages our minds, which is a scientific falsehood. The concept of age-associated cognitive challenges acknowledges the biological complexity and personal hardships of cognitive dysfunction, but frames brain aging (and caregiving) as a demanding but nonetheless stimulating undertaking that poses "challenges" to individuals and families. One succumbs to a "disease," but can rise to a "challenge" and gain wisdom, such that being labeled becomes an opportunity to learn, grow, and give back rather than a form of public condemnation. In this framework, suffering can be an opportunity for personal transformation in the face of a natural process rather than an inexorable struggle against a villainous adversary. I am actively trying to integrate this concept into the stories of my patients.

AD leads to a loss of self → Brain aging creates a change in self

We owe it to those who have aging brains not to reduce their humanity to one organ. All of us constantly change across our life span, and the late stages of brain aging are part of that continuum. As one patient, an eighty-year-old woman diagnosed with probable Alzheimer's disease, said, "I'm fine . . . this must be normal, I guess, for my age."[5] Using a new metaphor can help us see the person in Alzheimer's rather than seeing Alzheimer's in the person. Such a view also highlights the important wisdom that we are not solitary selves. Our very personhood is always evolving and depends on our relationships with other people. As relationships evolve because of memory loss, they have the potential to become richer and deeper rather than poorer and shallower.

As it is now, people shun those with dementia. We warehouse our elderly in homes and further distance them with stigmatizing labels that treat them as anything but normal. In fact, a big problem in long-term-care facilities is that the cognitively healthy actively avoid the cognitively impaired. When we can face our future selves in those who are unfortunate enough to age neurologically faster than us, and summon up the strength to devote ourselves to caring for them and see them as aging human beings representing the human condition rather than diseased victims, we can come to a point of enhanced self-awareness about our development. Relating to individuals with memory problems can open up deeper relationships and can foster our own personal growth. It can also solidify and validate relationships at the end of life and enable us to celebrate the interdependency that we are blessed with as families.

Fighting a war on Alzheimer's → Accepting and adapting to our finitude

We are not at war with our aging brains and it is dangerous and deluded to think that there is a quick fix just around the corner. It is much better to strip away the adversarial metaphors of the AD myth and begin to accept and embrace our mortality as best we can. Doing so can enrich the time we spend with loved ones and can enable us to achieve more vibrant and fulfilling lives. We can still hope for future treatments for brain aging without making our loved ones "victims" in a "war."

Money should be spent on basic research on brain aging, but *just how much* should be judged by realistic understanding of the priorities that face us in the world today, and measured against other competing health priorities including caregiving and prevention. Besides lessening the need for control and conquest that defines Western medicine, an ecological perspective can place greater emphasis on prevention and public-health interventions and less on wasteful interventions at the end of life. It can also attune us to the resources our culture offers to assuage the death and dying process, namely, assisted-living facilities and hospice care.

My dad has Alzheimer's → My dad has what people used to call "Alzheimer's"

We know that no one ever "has" Alzheimer's, and that the label carries a severe social stigma. The old framework of AD is scientifically imprecise and socially harmful to our loved ones, and thus we should calibrate the language that we use with the scientific knowledge that we have. By making the choice not to allow yourself (or your loved one) to be brought into the medicalized myth of AD you can preserve your humanity, age with greater dignity, and add quality to your later years. Alzheimer's disease need not enter your household if you don't wish it to, and adding a qualifier ("My dad has what people *used to call* AD," "My mom has *probable* Alzheimer's," "I have *so-called* Alzheimer's") can distance the person you're talking about from the sterilizing generality of the disease framework.

Alzheimer's is a slow death → Aging persons can still be vital contributors

Aging is a project, a work of existential art, a story that one continues to write until one can write it no more—it does not end when one is diagnosed with Alzheimer's by a doctor. The stigma of AD is powerful. But it should not restrict persons whose brains are aging from finding meaningful roles for themselves.

In Cleveland, as you will learn, persons with memory challenges and even AD diagnoses are participating in programs with children. Brain aging changes a person—some more than others—but it does not remove them entirely from society. In fact, those with dementia can still give back to their communities. There is vigor in aging. There is life to be found in the process of dying.

The anthropologist Emily Martin has written that many individual voices working together can challenge the hegemony of medical categories and produce "a resounding chorus."[6] By committing to a new language of brain aging, we can transcend the dominant Alzheimer's myth and intervene in our conceptions of body and self in a more honest and humane way. If all of us speak and think differently about brain aging, mortality, and caring for our loved ones, we can begin to jointly author a new cultural narrative that can shape the way we age in the twenty-first century.

A man is always a teller of tales, he lives surrounded by his stories and the stories of others, he sees everything that happens to him through them; and he tries to live his life as if he were telling a story.
— JEAN-PAUL SARTRE

I am already transforming the language I use in my own practice and integrating the new framework I have offered with increasing success so far. I know that how we think and speak about dementia will be crucially important in determining how we care for persons who have aging brains, not to mention how we all care about our own brains and the brains of our younger generations. Changing the story of AD, and being mindful of the language we use to understand brain aging, will remove the stigma from aging and can improve the quality of our later years.

Together we can begin to shift our view of AD.

And changing the story starts with you.

Whatever you do, or dream you can, begin it. Boldness has genius and power and magic in it.
— JOHANN WOLFGANG VON GOETHE

CHAPTER ONE

A Gateway to the Future of Old Age

*Progress is impossible without change, and those who
cannot change their minds cannot change anything.*

—George Bernard Shaw

I remember a story I heard as an undergraduate at Brown University about Socrates sitting outside the gates of Athens, deep in thought. Before long, a man approached him and said, "I'm thinking about moving into Athens. Can you tell me what it is like to live here?"

Socrates replied, "I would be happy to tell you, but first you must tell me what it was like in your previous home city."

The man grimaced and said, "Oh, it was awful. The people stab you in the back, forsake you, and rob you of all you hold dear. I am not leaving any friends behind, only enemies."

Socrates frowned and spoke in a somber tone: "Well, I'm sorry to tell you that you will find the same thing here in Athens." The man hung his head as he proceeded through the city gates.

A short while later, a second stranger stopped to speak to Socrates and inquired, "I am considering moving here to Athens. Can you tell me what it is like to live here?"

Socrates looked at the man and again replied, "I would be happy to tell you, but first, would you please tell me what it was like in your previous home city?"

The man smiled and said, "Where I come from the people all work together and help each other. Kindness is ubiquitous, and you are never treated with anything but the utmost respect."

"Welcome to Athens," said a smiling Socrates. "You are sure to find the same thing here."

Just as Socrates was able to help the two travelers shape their own expectations of Athens, the medical community stands at the gateways of their patients' futures, assisting people with memory challenges and their families in developing a concept of what to expect as they age. Many elderly patients come to their doctors harboring fear, terror, and angst about their memory loss that are generated from the public myth we have of Alzheimer's disease, which remains largely negative and simplistic. When it is not misunderstood completely, with talk of people "fading away" and "losing themselves," AD is seen through the prism of a war against a disease that attacks our brains late in life. Too often the emotion it evokes is fear, and not the empathy it deserves.

> ### THE SCARLET AD
>
> **"Can it be that the term 'Alzheimer's' has a connotation similar to the 'Scarlet Letter' or 'Black Plague'? Is it even more embarrassing than a sexual disease?"**
>
> —written by a woman diagnosed with Alzheimer's[1]

This preconceived terror that patients have about their memory loss is too often validated by their doctors, and the manner in which the diagnosis is communicated can be a devastating experience for persons and their families. Delivered without proper subtlety, the "Alzheimer's" label ushers in beliefs, attitudes, cultural meanings, scientific inaccuracies, and narrow treatment options that negatively affect what a person expects of his final years. In consequence, millions of people approach old age expecting to become burdens to their families and to society as they "fade away" and "lose their selves" to a "disease." Sadly, this is becoming the dominant view of the aging process for millions of people around the world, particularly in countries influenced by the Western Enlightenment and dominated by concepts of autonomy and rationality. Eastern conceptions of enlightenment in the spiritual sense may offer us wiser perspectives of the aging process and the roles of elders.

Since my days at Brown, the story of Socrates at the gates of Athens has always stayed with me. Though it might seem audacious to question one of the greatest philosophers in Western civilization, I think we and the medical community must go beyond Socrates. After all, geriatricians are not value-neutral philosophers standing pat at the gates of human wellness—rather, we absorb what our patients tell us in the clinical setting and help them and their families deal with the brain-aging process and all the confusion and angst that accompany it.

As seniors experience cognitive decline, physicians may either apply the standard "Alzheimer's" label or help patients and their families face the challenge of their own brain aging more positively and proactively—this choice will ultimately produce the personal beliefs that patients and their families will carry with them into the final chapters of their lives. How medicine chooses to respond to the challenges set forth in this book will play a crucial role in determining whether our society can reimagine brain aging in a more salutary way that sends emerging elders down a path that reduces their suffering and shame. As of now, the standard myth feeds into an extremely negative and deterministic view that can be summed up in the popular image of "loss of self" and "the death that leaves the body behind." In addition, this view treats aging persons technically, as if they were computers with malfunctioning hardware, and leaves the caring process vague and undeveloped while implying that nothing will get better until a technological fix comes along.[2]

YOU'RE ONLY AS OLD AS YOU THINK YOU ARE

In a recent article in *The New York Times*, Gina Kolata wrote: "Rigorous studies are now showing that seeing, or hearing, gloomy nostrums about what it is like to be old can make people walk more slowly, hear and remember less well, and even affect their cardiovascular systems. Positive images of aging have the opposite effects. The constant message that old people are expected to be slow and weak and forgetful is not a reason for the full-blown frailty syndrome. But it may help push people along that path."[3]

THE MEDIA AND ALZHEIMER'S

The standard story about AD in your newspaper will go something like this: Alzheimer's disease is caused by degeneration of the brain and a loss of nerve cells due to many, mostly unknown, factors, some of which are genetic. By understanding genes, these stories say, we can come to learn about the chemical changes in proteins in the brains of affected persons, develop drugs to prevent the abnormal proteins from doing damage, and fix memory problems that devastate victims and their families.

This is the linear, technological, and expensive story of Alzheimer's disease that many of us have grown up with. Throw in movie star Rita Hayworth and former President Ronald Reagan—both affected by Alzheimer's disease—stir in Nobel Prize–seeking hubris, the heavy hand of the pharmaceutical industry, a dash of hype about biotechnology, and a dollop of Washington politics, and we have developed an all-too-tragic and reductionistic narrative that dominates our hearts and minds. It is a story that medical professionals—myself included—have been telling to a terrified public for decades.

There are certain fundamental flaws in this story. All you thought you knew about AD needs to be reevaluated and challenged, and with it, our complete approach to aging. As someone who has dedicated his life to caring for patients in the AD field, I'm ready to put my integrity on the line in *The Myth of Alzheimer's*.

RESISTING THE MEDICALIZATION OF BRAIN AGING

As a longtime clinician, I can say that any dementia is a misfortune and a profoundly disconcerting one to persons and their families, and even to the doctors who care for aging persons.

> *Dementia* is a nonspecific blanket term that encompasses many processes that occur during the life span, even in children and young adults. There are many types of dementia, among which Alzheimer's disease is thought to be the most prevalent. Some other types are vascular

dementia, Lewy body dementia, frontal lobe dementia, Pick's disease, Parkinson's disease, Huntington's disease, and Creutzfeldt-Jakob disease.

I wish to suggest that both our perspective on brain aging and how we treat patients might be less distressing if we could give persons and their families the choice to see AD not as a loss of self wrought by a disease, but as a *change in self* that is not so unlike many others a person undergoes in various other life stages; not as a *war*, but as a natural stage of life that introduces challenges and offers opportunities for families to grow closer as they recognize the interdependency with others and embrace the opportunity for closeness in the face of cognitive loss. The effects of dementia *do* damage the awareness of one's identity and can be serious, troubling, and tragic. People may eventually lose some of their essential qualities, like communication. But these alterations in personhood give us little grounds for saying that an identity has been destroyed or lost, and certainly don't provide justification for ceasing to understand, engage, and include them in our own lives or in our society. Dementia changes selfhood but it does not erase it altogether or create non-persons who are shells of themselves. As Tom Kitwood, a pioneer in dementia care, once wrote, the perceived loss of self is not linked exclusively to the progress of the disease, but results from us projecting hopelessness and confusion onto people with dementia and failing to take time to engage them, understand their needs, perceive aging as part of the human condition, and reintegrate aging persons into our lives.[4]

MEDICALIZATION

Medicalization is a major trend that has taken place since the Enlightenment in which medicine and its scientific models, frameworks, and institutions have come to exercise judgment and influence over areas of our lives not previously considered medical. For instance, childbirths were not always carried out in hospitals, they were carried out in homes; nor were processes such as sexual dysfunction, hyperactivity, or circumcision previously considered primarily medical issues. Over the years, these and an increasing number of everyday practices have been caught in the net of medicalization and given narrowly scientific frameworks. We now have rigorous labor standards for pregnant women, pills to treat impotence and ADHD, and circumcision is an unquestioned hospital procedure for 80 percent of American families.[5] Those are the stories that shape our reality, some for better, some for worse.

> The "Alzheimerization" of dementia . . . has served to impede the process of cultural transformation.[6]
>
> —TOM KITWOOD

Brain aging hasn't always been a disease called Alzheimer's, and elderly persons haven't always beaten down their doctors' doors requesting that their brain aging be diagnosed as a disease and demanding pharmaceutical treatments and cures. Indeed, before our highly medicalized era, the story of brain aging has been told in many ways. *Dementia*, which has its origins in Latin and means "out of one's mind," was long ago used to identify various dissidents and deviants, especially older women who were castigated as witches when they began to show signs of mental decline.

The story has evolved throughout history. Aging men and women who lived in the nineteenth century would have been subjected to a story that told them their cognitive decline was owed to an ever-decreasing supply of vital energy that had dissipated since birth, and that their brains were simply growing cold, dry, and hard in the absence of an élan vital.[7] And as recent as the last century, dementia was actually associated with moral degeneration—namely, drinking, sexual excess, and masturbation. We are the first human beings to think of brain aging itself as a (tragic) neurological disease that can be repaired.

LESSONS FROM THE EAST

The loss of cognitive functioning that we experience as we age can be framed in a much more sympathetic way than we do in the rationally minded West. Although I am not a formally practicing Buddhist, I draw much wisdom from the Buddha's teachings and have, over the years, tried to integrate this wisdom into my clinical care. In particular, the Buddhist precept that life is like a flame has always evoked powerful sentiments in me.

*I . . . now see my reluctance to apply the term
Alzheimer's to my father as a way of protecting the
specificity of Earl Franzen from the generality of a
named condition.*[8]

—JONATHAN FRANZEN

As someone who has observed the aging and dying process in my patients, I know that the flame of a cognitively affected person's life is not ex-
tinguished by the dysfunction of the brain or the acquisition of a disease
label, but wanes as the individual slowly disconnects from the past, becomes unconcerned with the future, and lives only in a constant present.
The flame of personhood is always there.

Because our standard one-hundred-year-old medicalized myth of
Alzheimer's causes us to interpret the waning period of a person's cognitive

A STORY FROM MY PRACTICE

One of my patients was a former NFL star who had Alzheimer's and
Parkinson's disease symptoms. Though I was expecting a big, bruising,
aggressive man to come ambling into the clinic, I was surprised to be in
the presence of a quiet and peaceful man who was quite charming. Many
people fear that their loved ones will become aggressive or violent as their
dementia progresses, and this can be the case in some instances; but
dementia can also mollify individuals as they age and can potentially draw
them closer to a state of internal calm—even those who made a living out
of smashing into opponents! Whether a person with dementia exaggerates
their worst features or their best often depends on the circumstances they
are in, and especially on the type of caregiver they have. The former NFL
star had a wife who was a loyal and attentive caregiver. She viewed her
husband's condition as an opportunity to enrich and deepen their
relationship on different terms, and did her best to create an environment
that would best accommodate and stimulate her husband.

vitality as a tragic loss of self, we reflexively impose suffering and woe onto loved ones who are succumbing to the neurodegenerative process when they may actually be moving closer to a state of inward calm and simplicity. Families often fail to find redemption and meaning in the gradually changing state of their loved one. We change in every life stage, and progressive dementia actually creates the opportunity—difficult as it is—to deepen relationships and re-embrace a familial interdependency that our fast-paced lives often fracture. This is especially true for those of us with parents who are declining. Their reversion to a less functional state inverts the relationship we've had with them for our whole lives. It creates an interdependency that may not have existed before, an opportunity to return kindness, compassion, and warmth to our parents in their time of need. And if our relationship was strained, late-stage brain aging may even present an opportunity for reconciliation and redemption.

Elinor Fuchs, a professor of drama at Yale and one of my colleagues, has written a book called *Making an Exit,* about her mother, Lil, who had Alzheimer's. An indomitable and ambitious woman, Lil had damaged her relationship with her daughter through her career-driven style of living—so much that Elinor avoided her through her college years. However, as Lil's dementia progressed after her Alzheimer's diagnosis, the relationship between her and Elinor was transformed, with Elinor relishing the role of becoming her "mother's mother," and Lil connecting with her daughter at a level of intimacy achieved through the simplicity of her disintegrating language. When I spoke to Elinor at an Alzheimer's conference in the spring of 2007, she gave me a signed copy of her book and pointed out a quote on the back cover about her mother that expressed that "the last ten years, they were our best."

Indeed, watching a loved one decline is tragic, but, as I have seen time and time again with my patients, and even with my colleagues, within tragedy there is also opportunity for personal growth, warmth, and humor. Without speech there can still be touch and smiles. Without deep substantive conversation, you can still learn much about yourself in relation to the person with dementia. And, most important, without a pharmacological fix for brain aging, there can still be hope. Judith Levine, an author from Brooklyn who wrote a book about her father's dementia called *Do You Remember Me?*, once wrote this note to me after seeing me quoted in a *New York Times* article in which I expressed skepticism about current Alzheimer's drugs: "I was excited to see your name in the *Times,* finally going public about what so many of us already knew about AD drugs. Much of the response implies that the docs who doubt drugs are robbing sufferers and their families of hope. My own reaction was just the opposite: for the first time since my father was diagnosed twelve years ago, I feel hopeful that we may start to think and act differently about dementia."

> *Expect people to do better than they are;*
> *it helps them to become better;*
> *but don't be disappointed when they are not;*
> *it helps them to keep trying.*
>
> —UNKNOWN

THE POWER OF CHOICE

Indeed, there are an infinite number of stories that can be told about brain aging. A lovely counterexample to the Alzheimer's myth was written by my friend Ann Davidson, who has published two books about caring for her husband, Julian, a former Stanford professor who was affected by dementia and received a diagnosis of probable Alzheimer's. Her first book, *Alzheimer's: A Love Story,* recounted one year in her role as a caregiver. Ann told me she had to work very hard to get "love story" in the title because her publisher initially resisted the pairing of love and Alzheimer's disease. Ann's argument was that it is not necessary that tragedy be the lens through which we view cognitive decline. Instead of seeing her husband's condition as a loss of self that created a shell of a man and endless bereavement for her, she wanted to grow closer to him by embracing the interdependency caused by cognitive challenges. In her second book, *A Curious Kind of Widow,* which covers her caregiving experience in even greater detail, Ann writes: "During that first year after the diagnosis, in a hypnosis session with a psychiatrist, an insight came. As I lay stiff with anxiety on the doctor's couch, that wise man asked me what I wanted. Suddenly, a flash appeared: I wanted to 'go down' in a spirit of love, not fear and anger, no matter what happened."[9]

Ann and Julian's journey was still a great struggle, but one that was defined by emotional connection and happy, joyful times. Even when her husband's decline necessitated that he be placed in assisted living, he and Ann would still share quality time together—walking outdoors, listening to music, holding hands—and Julian managed to maintain a circle of friends and to volunteer at a local food bank. Ann's choice to go down in a spirit of love never faltered. Her story of love prevailed over the myth of AD.

STORIES FROM MY PRACTICE

A former patient of mine still sends me letters and postcards from the various locations she visits all over the world. In the past few years I've received postcards from Italy, Greece, Macedonia, Scotland, Australia, Thailand, and Japan. She has a progressive aphasia, meaning that she has lost nearly all abilities of speech and expression. Nevertheless, she and her husband have continued to travel the world doing what they love most, and have maintained a high quality of life by embarking on periodic journeys that expand their horizons and challenge them to adapt to new and novel situations. These trips have helped them both stay cognitively vital, and have enriched their relationship during what could otherwise be a period of slow, inexorable decline.

Another of my patients—a famous physicist—has a progressive dementia, but has continued to visit his colleagues in academia throughout the course of his brain aging. Staying connected helps him maintain a sense of belonging, as well as a sense of pride in his professional accomplishments. In his career, my patient had discovered a "constant"—a law of nature that became known throughout the world. Whereas my globe-trotting patient maintained quality of life through world travel, my physicist patient seemed to draw strength from the stability of his relationships with former colleagues. The lesson from these stories is simple: One of the keys to successful aging is to do what you love for as long as you can.

MY DEMOCRATIC APPROACH TO AGING

This book emphasizes choice—your choice. As with Ann and Julian, the story that you and your loved ones live by as you age is entirely yours to choose, and need not be the standard myth that is given to most of us by our doctors and informed by the fears and insecurities of society. Choice is paramount in any democratic culture, and an important aspect of quality of life. When we abdicate our democratic responsibility, we risk exposing ourselves to the tyranny of those who hold power over us. The same holds true in medicine: When we give too much power and responsibility to our doctors, we risk disempowering ourselves and limiting the story that we and our loved ones come to live by. It is not surprising that Plato, when describing his utopian Republic, emphasized that physicians would be limited in the power they held over the populace. The biomedical view of Alzheimer's disease is the dominant framework in our world today. But it need not dominate your life—we can make the choice to reframe the way we age.

DOES EMPOWERMENT HAVE COGNITIVE BENEFITS?

The Whitehall II study undertaken by British researcher Joan M. Griffin and colleagues revealed that elderly women who reported having less control in their lives had higher rates of cardiovascular disease and mental illness.[10]

The framework—or story—that we choose will have a significant impact on our sense of self-identity and well-being. The distancing, reductionist language of AD that forms our standard view divides persons with Alzheimer's and ourselves into separate categories of "us" and "them" and precludes the possibility of brain aging being a love story.

Remember, some decline of our brains over time is an invariable, some might say essential, aspect of who we are as mortal human beings; *cognitive decline actually validates that each of us is a living person, not that we are ceasing to be one.* Besides, contrary to those of my colleagues who wish to reduce humans to their brains (or even their neuroactive genes), I believe with all my heart that human beings are more than the sum of their cognitive equipment. As the philosopher Mary Midgley says: "People sometimes say that the human brain is the most complex item in the universe. But the whole person of whom that brain is part is necessarily a much more complex item than the brain alone."[11] No matter the decline in our cognitive functioning we still retain our humanity, and that humanity can still be engaged and loved even under the harshest changing circumstances: There is never a *"loss of self,"* only a *"change in self."*

And even in death, a loved one still retains their vitality through the stories we tell in their memory.

STORY—THE INSTRUMENT OF CHANGE

The story of AD can be reframed, and, as Ann Davidson's, Elinor Fuchs's, and Judith Levine's stories illustrate, the choice to do so is ours. The power of the Alzheimer's myth will begin to diminish when each of us starts to change the language we use to talk about brain aging. We must think and act in a more balanced manner, and less in terms of ambush, warfare, disease categories, losing and winning, the destruction of self-hood, and a bio–arms race. Humans and their aging brains are not at war. Persons with dementia are not a separate species from the rest of us. Rather, we are all engaged in the process of aging, and as we undergo this admittedly difficult process we have within us the potential for considerable wisdom, self-knowledge, and emotional connectivity.

THE JOURNEY OF ILLNESS

Anne Hunsaker Hawkins, a specialist in the Medical Humanities movement, has written a seminal book called *Reconstructing Illness: Studies in Pathography*. In it, she describes how illness-inspired writing and storytelling has proliferated in the last several decades, and that whether people are writing about their experience of AIDS, autism, bulimia, cancer, schizophrenia, stroke, or Alzheimer's disease, most people tend to choose archetypal narratives such as journey and rebirth to make sense of their condition. These narrative reconstructions often undercut the cultural myths prescribed by our society and help persons obtain answers to why they became ill, what illness means in the larger context of their lives, and how a new story can help accommodate the significant challenges that their illness brings and lead to new insight, meaning, and purpose. Anne believes that the process of writing and reframing illness is a profoundly healing experience.

CHANGING THE STORY

In Japan there are efforts under way to change the diagnostic terminology for persons labeled with mental illnesses associated with aging. The current label given to persons with dementia, *chihou,* is a compound word, with *chi* meaning "foolish and losing one's reason," and *hou* meaning "stupid and absent of mind." Several Japanese colleagues have told me that this connotation is often perceived as an insult, and that many people given a *chihou* diagnosis are often, quite understandably, ashamed and deeply resentful. The severe stigma has created the need for a new label. Professionals in the field have proposed that the new label be *ninchishou. Ninchishou* is also a compound word, with *ninchi* meaning "cognition," or "awareness," and *shou* meaning "dispositions," "symptoms," or "challenges"—roughly translating to "awareness of cognitive symptoms."

In 2005, Japan's Ministry of Health, Labor, and Welfare posted the intent, purpose, and related information of changing the name for dementia on their Web site and invited opinions from the public.

Ninchishou emerged as the victor.

The purpose of instituting this new terminology is that a patient given the label will better be able to reconcile their condition and adapt to it without feeling themselves to be fools. Likewise, such a semantic adaptation may lessen the tendency to ostracize aging persons, and may help communities embrace the elderly and see the person rather than the dementia. This is conceptual reframing at its best: Modify the label, change the story patients and their families find themselves a part of, and improve quality of life without compromising clinical care. Most important, change was brought about democratically by the Japanese people rather than just by the medical community. Precedent has been set for the end of the Alzheimer's myth, and we too can reject and replace the corrupted cultural myth of AD with a more humane and empathetic story that helps aging persons and their families.

To those who question whether changing words can really have a neurological impact, consider this: As a neuroscientist, I can tell you that every time you hear the word *Alzheimer's,* it affects your brain. The word triggers certain neural circuits that give access to our inner lexicon of words and meanings. Words that are loaded with powerful emotions (*Alzheimer's disease, death, terror, fear,* and so on) affect the brain in more powerful ways, and can even induce physiological changes in the brain, such as the release of stress hormones that may be damaging to neurons. Can precluding such changes by using different words help neurons survive? Maybe. But even in the event that they don't make a direct impact on the molecular level, different words and concepts can still assist people and families in adapting to their condition. The Japanese government wouldn't be spending so much money on developing a new terminology if words were only words.

WHY WE NEED TO ACT NOW

Today 25 million people around the world (and five million Americans) are said to be affected by Alzheimer's disease at immeasurable costs that have been estimated at $250 billion a year.[12] In the next decade, as members of the baby boom generation advance into their sixties, they will constitute the largest elderly population in our country's history. By the year 2030, it is estimated that nearly one-fifth (70 million) of the American population will be sixty-five or older, with average life expectancy being approximately 77.5 years for men and eighty-three for women.[13] And in 2040, it is estimated that there will be 40 million people aged eighty-five or older.[14] The demographic is even more profound in the developing world, which has large populations with increasing numbers of people who are living to an older age as modernization occurs. India and China already constitute the largest-ever populations of persons with dementia, and the developing world as a whole will comprise two-thirds of the worldwide Alzheimer's population. To put this in perspective, in the coming years, a new person will be diagnosed with AD every eleven seconds—unless we, like the Japanese, stop applying the label and imagine better stories to tell about the human condition.

As medicine continues to advance in its ability to treat such conditions as cardiovascular disease, which have largely affected the elderly population, people will live longer. And as people live longer, there will be unprecedented numbers of people in the later stages of brain aging. The number of Americans to be diagnosed with Alzheimer's disease is projected to reach 14 million by 2050 at a cost of well over $300 billion a year. The organization Alzheimer's Disease International (ADI) estimates the number of people worldwide to exceed 80 million.[15] Do we want a great number of these memory-challenged individuals, including ourselves, to live the sunset of their lives in fear with a stigmatizing disease label, as is already the case with millions around the world? Do we want to keep separating ourselves and our aging loved ones into categories of us and them?

Or would we rather take a more positive, humanistic approach to reassure them that most age-related memory loss and other functional slowdowns are normal components of aging that do not necessitate a disease label—that families and communities can take care of them rather than devaluing them? Would it not be better to believe that persons with cognitive challenges can still be vital human beings with high quality of life who can contribute to the social good and remain integral members of our families and communities, even with the apparent ravages of their memory loss? This is the story I am creating for my patients in Cleveland, where several persons with diagnosed dementia are volunteering as reading mentors in a local charter school that my wife and I created, and participating in art and narrative therapies that integrate them into the community and honor the personhood still remaining in each individual.

AND YOU WERE EXPECTING . . . ?

A study in 2004 showed that of eighty-eight people with mild to moderate dementia, 67 percent of persons diagnosed with dementia claimed they enjoyed a "very good" or "good" quality of life, while only 15 percent reported having a "bad" quality of life. For those who answered in the affirmative, good quality of life was generally associated with meaningful contact with others and the sense of being useful in a social context. Besides pointing out crucial elements of quality of life that we should all strive for, this study lends no support to the supposition that dementia is necessarily a state of dreadful suffering or a disaster without consolation, as so many assume.

CAN A BRAIN-AGING FRAMEWORK TRULY PREVAIL?

One of my colleagues has questioned me by sharing the story of a sixty-six-year-old mother of three who expressed that she wanted to kill her husband and confessed to feeling "stupid" and being unable to do anything for her family. He told me that this woman had a history of progressive cognitive loss, and that routine neuroimaging and blood tests previously detected no specific signs of other dementias. In other words, her story was entirely consistent with a diagnosis of Alzheimer's disease. Can we truly refer to this woman's case as normal aging? my colleague has asked me.

Clearly when brain aging hits earlier than we expect it to, and especially when it features prominent behavioral symptoms such as aggressiveness and suicidal thoughts, it is impossible to call a person's situation normal. Statistically speaking, it is not normal to be so demented at sixty-six, whereas the onset of some dementia in one's eighties, nineties, or beyond is more or less the normal expectation. I use the word *normal* because our bodies and minds, which have evolved over millions of years, have been optimized to ensure the proliferation and survival of our species rather than an extended life span for individuals. Thus, the onset of age-related conditions such as brain aging appears to be part of the "normal" sequence of events that takes place after we have reached an age when we can no longer reproduce and fulfill our evolutionary purpose.[16] It would actually be quite abnormal for someone *not* to have increasing memory challenges in their seventies, eighties, and beyond.

To return to my colleague's patient, I am willing to agree that we might justifiably refer to this woman's condition as a disease, or at least as abnormal because it exists outside the normal range of pathology that we would expect for someone her age. However, the essential question is: Do we practically need to consider her case and ones similar to it as diseases? Does that sort of approach contribute to her care or detract from it?

For some families, the standard disease model is necessary and comforting, but, as I've seen in my practice, others who are disturbed by disease labels are receptive to choosing more open-minded ways of approaching the situation. Let's imagine ourselves in the place of the woman's clinician. You cannot cure her disease; you cannot adequately treat her disease; you can only offer a probable diagnosis of her disease as being Alzheimer's. However, what you *can* influence is the story that she and her family enter into. Say that we *do* label this woman with "Alzheimer's disease" and introduce this culturally powerful story into her life. In my clinical experience, this lends justification to her feelings of stupidity and uselessness, lowers expectations for her, and gives her more reason to be upset, aggressive, and disdainful. The story of the disease can become self-fulfilling and exacerbate an already-challenging situation.

On the other hand, to take time to sit and talk with this woman and her family and tell them that all of the tests indicate that she is prematurely aging, but that she and her family can adapt to her changing circumstances, frames her decline in a much different light. It can normalize her hardships and assuage her feelings of victimization and hopelessness. It can pose challenges to her and her family instead of implying a tragic decline with no redemption. We can still pursue every treatment option available—including drugs— while shaping a gentler and more holistic brain-aging narrative for the patient and her family if they choose to go beyond the standard myth of Alzheimer's.

A few years ago, Michael J. Fox wrote an autobiography called *Lucky Man*, detailing his early-onset Parkinson's disease and demonstrating how reframing one's life story to incorporate illness can lead to greater meaning. Fox refers to himself not as a victim but as a "lucky man" for getting Parkinson's, because the condition transformed his life in positive ways as he adapted to his physical disability. Fox's story shows us that while every human malady has a biological basis, it is also socially constructed, and that the latter dimension helps us interpret and behave toward the biological condition. The dominance of the Alzheimer's disease model as a guiding framework for aging persons precludes more enlightened thinking about the process of our own aging. *Again, the way we choose to frame brain aging is crucial.*

In order for the boomer generation to meet the unprecedented challenges of our increasingly aging society, we must reflect on our current paradigms of care for people of advanced age and our attitudes about aging and mortality. We must consider how we can promote quality of life for men and women in an effective and cost-effective way as we age and experience memory loss. Baby boomers will not age as their parents did. We will be more reflective about our long decline and receptive to new ways of thinking about our bodies and our minds that challenge formally dominant models. *The Myth of Alzheimer's* is part of a new movement toward redefining our understanding of aging.

SIZING UP THE BOOMERS

- 76.9 million is the estimated number of baby boomers in the U.S.

- 26.8 percent of the nation's population are baby boomers.

- 51 percent of boomers are women.

- $45,654 is the average annual spending by boomer households.

- 12.6 percent of boomers have never married.

- 88.8 percent of boomers completed high school.

- 28.5 percent of boomers have a bachelor's degree or higher.

- Nine states (California, Florida, Illinois, Michigan, New Jersey, New York, Ohio, Pennsylvania, and Texas) are where more than half of all boomers live.

Source: MetLife Mature Market Institute

THE WISDOM OF OPRAH: A LOOK BACK AND WAY FORWARD

In the 1980s, I, like many of my colleagues, had an earnest hope that AD was a biological disease that could be significantly ameliorated through the development of drugs. In fact, I remember sitting on the stage of Oprah Winfrey's show in the mid-1980s to share important developments in my Alzheimer's research at Johns Hopkins University. I told a national television audience what I now consider to be the standard story of AD. The show's producers had recruited me as an expert on Alzheimer's, and I was asked to interview several individuals whose lives had been affected by the disease. One was a professional ballerina whose neurosurgeon husband had died of AD; another was an African-American woman who had gotten separated from her family in New York City for three days and was cared for by a homeless community on the streets.

Although even then I harbored some reservations about the scientific precision of our classification of Alzheimer's disease, I played my customary role well, speaking about AD with a measured confidence. No fewer than three times did Oprah, a persistent interviewer, ask me to clarify how AD isn't merely a form of senility. *Senility,* I said, is an imprecise lay word, whereas Alzheimer's disease has a clear medical definition that classifies a biological pathology: It is a neurodegenerative disease that causes neuronal loss and atrophy.

Looking back on that interview, I am impressed at Oprah's prescient observations about the social construction of AD. At the time, I assumed she was unfamiliar with the latest thinking about dementia. In hindsight, she was a step ahead of me. Perhaps Oprah was asking me to get beyond the hype of the disease myth and contemplate what two decades later has become the central question surrounding AD: *Should biomedical disease labels with frightening cultural meanings be used to describe a condition that might otherwise be considered variable human brain aging?*

ACCEPTING THE LIMITS OF SCIENCE

Science has collected much data on the brain and frequent claims are made for dramatic leaps in understanding how the brain processes information. Yet we really do not know how the brain works, how thoughts are produced, and why we are conscious of our own cognition. Moreover, only baby steps have been made in mitigating the symptoms of memory loss, which affect millions of families worldwide. Our fixation on biomedical research couches Alzheimer's disease in purely mechanical and molecular terms and dumps all our resources into the inexorable search for a cure. The fact is: Brain aging is not something that can be cured. The cognitive decline that accompanies old age is unavoidable, but we can find ways to make sure these cognitive challenges don't decrease our overall effectiveness or quality of life.

I am not suggesting that therapeutic discoveries will never emerge. In fact, I have no doubt that more effective therapies can be developed, but the questions are: How powerful will these therapies be, when will they arrive, how expensive will they be, and at what opportunity costs to society? Our resources and our hope are being overinvested in the search for a far-off cure when, really, the genuine and effective answers lie within ourselves, and in our ability to care for one another.

That said, if my father, mother, or wife were to develop disabling cognitive problems, I would love for a magic bullet to appear. But whether or not a cure does appear to save the day, I would, like Ann Davidson, choose to "go down" in a spirit of love, celebrating the life and the legacy my loved one has left, and hoping that my spirit of love would transform my fear, sadness, and anger and make caregiving easier and more meaningful. I would, like Ann, strive to be more fully present in my loved one's life and to enjoy the simple pleasures—holding hands, going on walks, listening to music, and eating meals. In this way, I would hope to rise to being a more caring individual in my relationship with them and not let the disease interfere with the evolution of our relationship. For it is in caring, and not technological prowess, that we can find the true hope in Alzheimer's disease.

At no time in the history of our species has an adaptation to aging and our mortality been more critical. There are not only more older people alive today with aging bodies and minds than ever before, but also more challenges to the adaptation of our species on a planet of finite resources. The Alzheimer's movement is a march-to-progress juggernaut: Give us enough time, people, and money, the line goes, and we will fix it. But after thirty years of research and tens of billions of dollars spent, we're not even close. In fact, our expensive genetic tests and neuroimaging devices have actually caused us to drift deeper into confusion and little closer to finding a cure. We are giving people false hope. Further investment might lead to the development of drugs that can ameliorate some of the negative effects of brain aging, but after thirty years of relative failure in drug development, shouldn't we begin to consider reallocating some of our resources into other avenues, for example: investing in educating people as to the preventive (behavioral) measures we can all take over the course of our life spans to avoid damage to our brains, and developing alternative therapies such as narrative-based, music, and touch interventions, or, on developing innovative caregiving practices for the patients and families who are adapting to memory challenges? The cultural myth hypes the cure. Our new story needs to have a greater emphasis on prevention and care.

In the chapters that follow, I will suggest de-emphasizing treatment with prescription drugs in favor of nonpharmacological interventions (mental, social, physical, and spiritual activities) that engage the whole aging person rather than treating their aging brain. I will advocate for public-health prevention measures that can treat the *causes* of brain aging and not merely its *effects*, as our current approach does. For instance, we must succeed in reducing environmental toxins such as lead and mercury in our homes, rivers, and parks that are responsible for producing neurological disease, particularly in young children, and we must also address the social contexts that subject many persons in our world to poverty, malnutrition, infection, trauma, hard labor, and mental lethargy that hasten cognitive decline.

I will articulate a plan for our cities to provide better care for aging persons and support their families. Further, I will strongly urge doctors to move away from the clinical usage of such labels as "Alzheimer's disease" and "Mild Cognitive Impairment" (MCI) with patients—or at least be more judicious in applying the labels and putting people in fixed categories. This will open up a new path along which families and their loved ones can age—a path of self-determination and hope.

THE PROBLEM OF MILD COGNITIVE IMPAIRMENT

Mild Cognitive Impairment (MCI) is a supposed precursor to AD that is alleged to exist along the continuum between normal aging and Alzheimer's. In other words, it is said to represent a gray area between normalcy and disease, which is difficult to define. As you would expect, this classification has met some resistance from clinicians, and the Alzheimer's pharmaceutical industry has been called into question for pushing for the formation of a new classificatory niche that expands potential drug consumers (and patients) by extending pathology onto those who may be undergoing basic brain aging. There has even been talk of promoting a category called pre-MCI! The label is particularly worrisome when you consider its import into other cultures. For example, one Chinese opinion leader has translated the term Mild Cognitive Impairment into Chinese and back into English as "loss of wisdom." The stigmatization and despair such a label could cause is very worrying indeed.

Many years ago, a vigorous older patient of mine, a professional actress, told me that old age had been a source of empowerment for her. "Aging doesn't tame you," she said during one of her appointments. "It creates the opportunity to take more risk."

THE POWER OF STORIES: A NARRATIVE APPROACH TO ENDING ALZHEIMER'S

By changing the way we think about Alzheimer's, we change the story we tell about our aging brains. That matters because stories surround us, shape us, serve as the building blocks of our lives, and weave us into our human communities. As children, we are told simple tales from which we draw lessons about the world, and as we get older we advance to novels, textbooks, myths, legends, fables, gospels, tragedies, dramas, comedies, songs, television shows, and films that offer stories with more complex moral and historical themes that we integrate into the fabric of our character.[17]

Even in our day-to-day lives stories are ubiquitous, appearing in news-papers, on television, on the Internet, surfacing in conversations with friends, in e-mails and cell phone discussions, and even cropping up in our inner monologues and daydreams. The stories most meaningful to us are the ones that give shape to our values and beliefs, and form cognitive frames that help us sort out a complex world that might otherwise over-whelm us. As the philosopher Alasdair MacIntyre has written in his book *After Virtue,* humans create their sense of what matters by referring con-sciously or unconsciously to the stories they have learned: "I can only an-swer the question 'What am I to do?' if I can answer the prior question 'Of what story or stories do I find myself a part?' "[18] Language is the mediating factor that constitutes our self, and we have an instinctive desire to orga-nize our experiences into narrative form.

One reason I find Alzheimer's disease so disturbing is because its de-scription comprises a powerful story that generates tremendous fear, angst, and social stigmatization for the millions diagnosed with AD and for mil-lions more of us who are aging. There is a difference between telling some-one that her brain is aging and helping to incorporate her into her community, and telling her that she has an underlying progressive degener-ative brain "disease" called Alzheimer's and applying a label that could os-tracize her. The story that the doctor chooses will doubtlessly shape the narrative arc of that person's life; it is a story that can even write a person out of the community. As the sociologist Erving Goffman has written, a stigmatized person who is branded with a feared or hated label is one who has lost his or her wholeness in society's eyes: "He is reduced in our minds from a whole and usual person to a tainted, discounted one."[19]

THE AD LABEL CAN DISABLE

I once had a very bright and charismatic patient who was adamant that she would commit suicide if it turned out that she had Alzheimer's disease. Some people come to me holding this extreme position, because the AD label has a way of driving suicidal thoughts. In this woman's case, and in each such instance I encounter in my practice, I attempted to persuade her to think more positively about the trajectory of her condition, and emphasized the variability of the clinical course of brain aging. I reminded her that even if the worst-case scenario played out and she declined quickly, she might become more serene and at peace with her condition, losing the desire to commit suicide in the process. There was always the chance that her decline would not be steep, and that she would be able to draw great meaning, purpose, and fulfillment from her later years.

Nancy Waxler, an anthropologist who helped develop social labeling theory, has shown that the socially stigmatizing labels we use in Western industrialized countries often prolong and exacerbate illness.[20] For instance, she found that in modern societies, expectations and beliefs about mental illness serve largely to alienate schizophrenic patients from their normal roles and thus to prolong illness. In contrast, nonbiomedical beliefs and practices held in nonindustrial societies encouraged shorter-term illness and a quicker return to normality. From my own limited personal experience dealing with worker's compensation (assessing injuries at work that limit a person's ability to do a job), I am convinced that if there is an economic advantage to being labeled with a neurological condition, people will remain disabled longer. That is the self-fulfilling power of labels.

I am writing this book for one simple reason: to empower readers to stand up to the dominant, stigmatizing biological myth of Alzheimer's that scientists like myself, with more than a little help from the drug companies and others with financial and personal interests, have unleashed on individual lives, and to reframe the way we know and experience our aging selves. Some welcome the Alzheimer's label, since it can both mobilize resources and absolve individuals of blame for the deterioration of mental functioning. I believe that this same result can be accomplished by changing the way we approach brain aging. We can provide quality care and resources for our aging elders without stigmatizing them with a scientifically imprecise and socially damaging disease. We don't need to label someone just because it is demanded by a health insurance billing code or a politician's budget.

Our scientific understanding of Alzheimer's disease becomes more complicated every day. The story of brain aging is ultimately your own story to tell, not mine, not your doctor's, and certainly not the self-interested pharmaceutical companies or research institutions that capitalize on our biological classification of AD as a disease. *Alzheimer's* has been the way Western culture has described brain aging for the past one hundred years. By taking that myth apart from a biological, social, and historical perspective, I will show you that it doesn't need to be the dominant story in your life or the life of an aging family member.

> *Once you have removed all the dead language, the secondhand dogma, the truths that are not your own but other people's, the mottos, the slogans . . . the myths of your historical moment—once you have removed all that warps experience into a shape you do not recognize and do not believe in—what you are left with is something approximating the truth of your own conception.*
>
> —ZADIE SMITH

Changing the way we view things can change your life, and the story that you wish to live by as you age as a human being is very much in your power to choose. *If we can reframe the way we think, speak, and act toward our aging brains, and integrate new language, new psychosocial understandings, beliefs, attitudes, prevention measures, and treatment options into our biomedical paradigm of AD, we can reimagine the story of Alzheimer's disease and describe brain aging in a way that brings quality to people's latter years rather than adding distress and fear, and that better helps our society prepare for a challenging future.* A new therapeutic narrative can foster hope for the millions who are aging and fearing such age-related conditions as AD. As disruptive as the brain-aging process can be, it will never overshadow your humanity, strip away your dignity, or negate your own life story. Although our memory and recall capacity will inevitably deteriorate to one degree or another over time as we age due to age-associated physiological changes in the brain, the human hunger to be heard and respected—an instinct central to the human experience and often ignored by reductionistic biological medicine that looks only to treat malfunctioning organs—will never entirely vanish.

In writing this book, I want to help you overcome the fearsome story of Alzheimer's and deal with brain aging on your own terms, making sure the story of AD never overwhelms you or your family. I want your evolving story to be a piece of a larger societal movement in which we engage our moral imagination—the collective generative force of intellect, reason, feeling, and imagination—and begin to reconceptualize our attitudes and approach to death and dying. This book ultimately seeks to nurture the unfolding of *your story*. It is about overcoming your fear of Alzheimer's disease by gaining knowledge about brain aging, and learning to reframe a narrative for yourselves that will promote quality of life, cognitive vitality, and a sense of purpose and community as you age.

> *All sorrows can be borne if you put them into a story*
> *or tell a story about them.*
>
> —ISAK DINESEN

CHAPTER TWO

ALZHEIMER'S 101: TAMING THE SCIENTIFIC STORY OF AD

When a science appears to be slowing down and, despite the efforts of many energetic individuals, comes to a dead stop, the fault is often to be found in a certain basic concept that treats the subject too conventionally. Or the fault may lie in a terminology which, once introduced, is unconditionally approved and adopted by the great majority, and which is discarded with reluctance even by independent thinkers, and only as individuals in isolated cases.

—JOHANN WOLFGANG VON GOETHE

A few years ago, one of my colleagues in the Alzheimer's field who is a neuroscientist from a large university in Ohio pulled me aside at a conference and told me that he'd had enough of the AD myth.

"I feel guilty about being part of this entrenched social and political empire that is Alzheimer's disease," he told me. "We're doing such a disservice to people by making big promises about what Alzheimer's is and overselling what we can deliver. We've created a monster. I'm tired of being a part of that."

As the Alzheimer's myth has grown into a front-page issue in our culture, physicians have had to deal with the dilemma of facing patients who believe themselves to have a disease that can't be definitively diagnosed, much less treated or cured. Many of my colleagues have been unwilling to be honest publicly about our limited comprehension of brain aging, and the problematic and arbitrary nature of the labels we use. Part of this may stem from the fact that people have given their professional lives to fighting Alzheimer's and don't wish to concede that we haven't made the progress in diagnosing and treating the condition we would have hoped for in the last several decades. Their reluctance may also stem from the fact that the pharmaceutical industry has such powerful influence over many doctors, and the AD and MCI frameworks—stigma aside—help them sell drugs to millions of people.

FRONT ROW CENTER AT THE ALZHEIMER'S EMPIRE

Several years ago, I was invited to a fund-raiser gala in New York City hosted by the local Alzheimer's Association chapter. All around me at this opulent ten-thousand-dollar-a-table affair were industry executives, scientists, and consultants adorned in tuxedos and flowing evening gowns. I had been invited there as a guest of Forest Labs, a pharmaceutical company for which I consulted, which produced the Alzheimer's drug memantine.

After several speeches, the MC of the event stood before the roomful of wealthy donors and said quite resolutely, "We are going to find a cure for this disease someday! And that day is getting closer!" Inspired by this unqualified proclamation of hope, the donors on hand opened their pockets, raising hundreds of thousands of dollars for the Alzheimer's Association in one night. Did it occur to them that we don't know what "Alzheimer's disease" even is? Probably not. Hope often gets the better of common sense. And false hope is a better fund-raiser than realistic expectations. Organizations that comprise the AD empire thrive because the Alzheimer's myth is a cash cow that keeps on giving. Many of us in the field worry that the pursuit of truth has been eclipsed by the pursuit of raising funds.

There are a growing number of us who, as my colleague said, want to end the cruel reign of the Alzheimer's disease "monster" and ease the grip of fear it has on us. We want to empower you to see that although your brain will inevitably age as you grow older, creating challenges and difficulties for you and your family, you will never be stricken with a disease called Alzheimer's or become victim to some cognitive contagion. Changing the way we think and speak about our aging bodies can help us approach cognitive decline with greater wisdom.

> *Alzheimer's disease, as science seeks to grasp it, seems to slip through our fingers. The complex interactions of neurochemistry, genetics, environment, life story and personality all play a part in how individuals experience dementia. No single approach will explain everything.*[1]
> —HARRY CAYTON, NATIONAL DIRECTOR FOR PATIENTS AND THE PUBLIC, NATIONAL HEALTH SERVICE IN BRITAIN

ALZHEIMER'S 101

I must admit that the myth of Alzheimer's disease can be a monstrous one. It's no wonder people are afraid. After all, no one wants to lose themselves to such a horrific degenerative disease as AD. But we must first consider whether or not Alzheimer's is a disease. Surely our brains, just like our fragile bodies, fail us physiologically as we age: But how are we to know when this process ceases to be the normal trajectory of brain aging and starts being the work of a fearsome disease? Just how much forgetfulness in our daily lives does it take to qualify as a disease and how much can be chalked up to normal aging?

Despite the billions of dollars we've spent on research in the last several decades, not even the best scientists in the world have an answer to these questions. No one knows what the molecular event is that differentiates Alzheimer's from aging. Claims have been made, but, as is all too frequent with "breakthroughs," they have not been replicated by other scientists.

Remember, I am no stranger to the standard myth; I was trained to believe in it and have even helped develop it and spread it. I was once certain that AD would be a horror story with a happier ending. Now I'm not so sure. I think we've told the story all wrong, and I agree with my colleague that we have created a monster in the process that needs to be tamed.

AN INTRODUCTION TO MEMORY

In our culture, we tend to visualize the brain as being a memory storage database, a personal hard drive onto which we load bits and bytes of experience, knowledge, and images. While this popular metaphor is helpful, memory is best thought of as a complex process rather than as a repository from which we extract information. This is because the process of storing memories is bound up with thought, emotion, and perception, and involves the interaction of multiple subsystems in the brain that work together in almost all situations involving the storage and recall of memory. In large part, our recall of memory takes place in narrative form; as others have said, we do not "store" experience on data, like a computer: We "story" it.[2]

We also do our remembering with more than our brains. Our bodies and their hormonal, muscular, and metabolic processes play a key role in supporting the brain. Perhaps the ultimate truth is that we rarely remember things without a social context in which those around us facilitate and influence our memory recall. Almost assuredly, anyone reading this book can count many people in their lives whom they draw on to remember specific information on their behalf: codes to bank accounts, phone numbers, relatives' birthdays, and family genealogy. We all store information in those around us—family, friends, coworkers—and when we lose these co-holders of information we often feel as if we've lost part of our external memory system. Memory is a social phenomenon often shared jointly with those closest to us. It cannot be reduced solely to our brains. Even so, for the purposes of studying AD, let's narrow our focus on the brain and look more deeply at the neural processes of memory.

Selection

Each waking moment of our lives we are barraged by endless information. Sensory stimulation streams in from our sense organs and enters our brains, which process the information, filtering out the great majority of it. What sticks is the information that, for emotional and contextual reasons, we remember. For instance, if we attend a one-hour lecture by Bill Gates, we may jot down notes of what was most significant to us. Even though Gates will have spoken thousands of words, we sift through his sentences, filter out the great majority, and commit to memory that which we deem essential. What we actually remember *sans* notes from the lecture, particularly days or months later, is remarkably limited. Needless to say, no one can remember every sensory aspect of our lived life (although those with photographic memory do well with visual images and sequences).

> *The existence of forgetting has never been proved: We only know that some things don't come to mind when we want them.*
> —FRIEDRICH NIETZSCHE

The variability in memory functions in so-called normal people is remarkable and yet all normal people function in life by compensating for weak areas (names of people) with strengths (visual imagery).

Neurons

As infants, we are born with many billions of neurons in our brains. Neurons—also more commonly called nerve cells—have a cell body, an axon, and dendrites, and they operate through the transmission of electrical impulses. These electrical signals, called action potentials, are caused by the flow of charged elements (such as sodium and potassium) across the boundaries of the cell, called a cell membrane. At the end of the long axon the cell releases chemicals called neurotransmitters that shuttle across the gaps in between neurons, called synapses, to stimulate chemical transmission and enhance neuronal firing or inhibit electrical activity in the dendrites of the receiving cell. This release of neurotransmitters at numerous dendrites enables neurons to link together synaptic connections with thousands of other neurons. These complex neural circuits, through processes science doesn't entirely comprehend, create and maintain our memories.

Storage

The process by which information is stored in neurons is poorly understood. For a memory to form, neurons must change their pattern of firing.

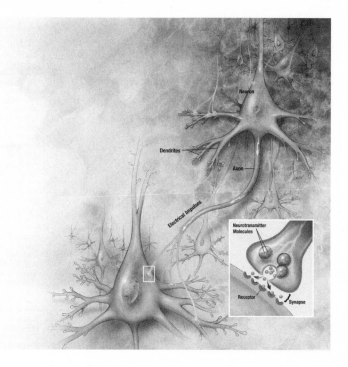

Figure 2. Diagram of a Neuron.   Courtesy of the National Institute on Aging, *Alzheimer's Disease: Unraveling the Mystery.*

One such pattern is called long-term potentiation, a process in which some synaptic connections are strengthened to enable nerve cells to remember and thus respond differently to future input or activity. Again, imagine watching Gates speak. Most of what he says is unconsciously filtered out, but you may write down several of his more profound statements that seem to resonate with you. After the lecture, to commit them to memory you need to concentrate on them and perhaps repeat the phrases again and again to try to remember how they are worded. This focusing of attention is increasing electrical activity in certain regions of your brain and releasing neurotransmitters between thousands of your synapses. This increased activity builds synaptic connections from neuron to neuron that ultimately solidify the statements in your mind and leave you more inclined to remember those statements in the future, if prompted. Not all things that you remember require conscious effort, however. In fact, our ability to control the memories that we store and those that we forget is quite limited.

LIVING IN THE NOW

Buddhism teaches a neurologically sound lesson: that we should all live in the moment. Two of the Buddha's teachings were:

"Do not dwell in the past, do not dream of the future, concentrate the mind on the present moment."

"The secret of health for both mind and body is not to mourn for the past, nor to worry about the future, but to live the present moment wisely and earnestly."

Indeed, whether you are meeting someone for the first time and trying to remember their name, or attempting to memorize facts that you read in the newspaper, paying attention in the present is extremely important for recalling memories later.

This is not the complete story. Our actual memories are constructed by groups of cells interacting together. There is no grandmother cell that has exclusive rights to retaining the memory of your grandmother. One important complex cluster of nerve cells is called the hippocampus. The hippocampus is a curved organ beneath the cortical layer of the brain in the temporal lobe (behind your ears), which derives its name from the Greek word for *seahorse*. When selected information streams in from your senses, the hippocampus, in ways we do not completely understand, converts some short-term memories into long-term ones. Damage to the hippocampus at any age impairs our ability to put information into a form that allows recall years later. Multiple factors like lack of oxygen to the brain, some infections, alcoholism, stress, depression, and normal aging itself are associated with loss of cells in the hippocampus. Additionally, the cholinergic basal forebrain, a cluster of nerve cells that I studied at Johns Hopkins which produces the transmitter acetylcholine, sends its axons to the hippocampus, and stimulates the structure with the neurotransmitter. When the cholinergic basal forebrain ceases to produce adequate levels of acetylcholine, it also affects the hippocampus and other brain regions, and thus our ability to learn and remember.

Recollection. The process of recollecting memories involves us engaging the information we've managed to store, usually in response to a cue. Formally

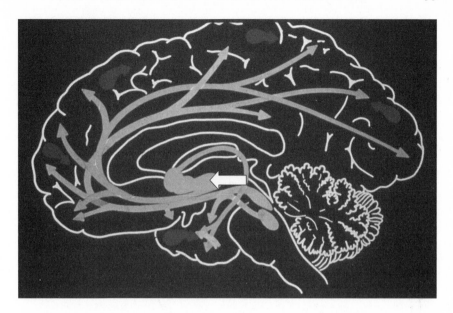

Figure 3. Cholinergic Basal Forebrain and Other Neuronal Populations Affected in Alzheimer's. Neurons in the cholinergic basal forebrain (indicated with the arrow) produce acetylcholine and send its axons to the hippocampus and elsewhere throughout the brain. Other cell populations shown on the diagram are also affected in aging and dementia.

speaking, recognition involves seeing a person, object, word, or sensation again and knowing you have experienced it before. Spontaneous recall means digging a memory out of the brain without a cue. However, memory does not work like a computer in that we do not simply double-click on a mouse and open a file in our minds. We engage memories creatively, bringing

---

LONDON ON THE MIND

A recent study looked at the hippocampi of taxi drivers in London, who commit to memory huge swaths of the famous city. Cabbies are expected to take a test called "The Knowledge," in which they must memorize nearly twenty thousand London streets and landmarks, as well as the quickest routes throughout the city. Investigators found that part of the hippocampus (the posterior hippocampus) is in fact larger in the taxi drivers than in the general public, and that the size of the hippocampus was positively associated with years of experience.[3]

our present perceptions, emotions, and thoughts into the recall process. For instance, after a couple drinks at an after-work cocktail party, someone might bring up Bill Gates and his unimaginable fortune (or his sometimes irritating operating system and business model). This activates the neural circuit you've formed about Gates, and you, realizing that you cannot recall his actual words, paraphrase a few of Gates's quotes, interspersing a few of your own words and ideas. Memory recall is contextual and bound up with emotions—thus, it is imperfect and fallible, as is the scientific understanding of how it all works.

CLASSIFYING MEMORY

There are many ways to classify memory, but most models agree on these types:

Episodic memory. Autobiographical facts, long-term memories (stories from one's childhood). Episodic memory is slow to develop in children and may be associated with the ability to tell stories. Failure to recall recent events is a hallmark of aging. Long-term episodic memories, for instance memories from one's childhood, are remarkably well preserved in older people, even those with cognitive challenges.

Semantic memory. Facts that stand alone from personal experience often associated with the meaning of specific words (the United States gained its independence in 1776; the definition of the word *democracy* is government by the people; the four Beatles were John, Paul, George, and Ringo). Semantic memory is often lumped together with episodic memory under the heading of "declarative memory"—a blanket term for memory that stores facts and personal experience rather than rote skills.

Procedural memory. How to complete motor tasks (remembering how to tie one's shoe, ride a bike, or play a guitar riff). Procedural memory is often beyond articulation; it is memory that is embodied: what we sometimes refer to as muscle memory. Imagine trying to explain to someone how to ride a bike: The action is easy enough to perform, but very difficult to articulate.

Working memory. Our short-term memory (remembering the phone number of the pizza place around the corner for fifteen seconds while you dial it on your phone). Working memory can be thought of like an Etch A Sketch: We jot down important information and then shake the slate clean moments after.

Implicit memory. The subtle implications that we remember without much voluntary cognition (you experience an aversion to a food that made you sick many years ago), also the déjà vu effect (you swear you remember seeing the black-haired woman in the grocery store before).

With Western culture placing such emphasis on the importance of cognition, many of us suffer from an almost neurotic fear of an inevitable decline in our ability to store and recall memories, particularly episodic and semantic memories that seem to be indispensable placeholders of our identity. In fact, in most surveys, nearly half of people over fifty report that their memory is abnormally impaired, with many worrying that this foreshadows a descent into Alzheimer's disease. As you will learn, over time a variety of factors—some genetic, some hormonal, some environmental, some related to the diminution of blood supply and glucose in the brain due to factors like diabetes or vascular problems—inevitably contribute to the dysfunction and sometimes death of neurons. This process occurs in all human beings to one degree or another as we age, and we gradually lose our visual acuity, our hearing, our sense of smell, and even basic mechanisms such as the ability to regulate the temperature of our bodies, and of course, our memory.

FORGET MEMORY

My colleague Anne Basting has written a book entitled *Forget Memory* (due for publication in 2008). The book acknowledges the fear of memory loss that is present in our culture but questions whether that fear makes the experience of the disease much worse than it needs to be. *Forget Memory* addresses that fear head-on and inspires us to imagine what the experience of memory loss might be like if fear wasn't our first and only reaction. How might our care system change? How might the lives of real people change? Our loved ones? Ourselves? I would highly recommend Anne's book, as she is someone who is challenging our conventional fears and presumptions about aging and memory loss in remarkably creative ways.

When this decline actually starts is an arbitrary distinction—some have proposed that brain aging begins after age twenty when we have the maximum amount of neurons in our brains, others implicate our peak fertility as the tipping point, while some profess that the decline of memory begins after age forty. In my opinion, the process of brain aging is best thought of as a continuum along which we all progress at different rates. As we move along this continuum, our ability to process, store, and recall information will inevitably be compromised, and memory loss will be positively associated with age. In some sense, we would all get Alzheimer's if we lived long enough. As you can imagine, along this continuum of brain aging, the lines among normal aging, AD, and MCI are not clearly defined. But that hasn't stopped scientists and advocacy organizations from trying to draw clear boundaries.

A STORY ABOUT MCI

I once had an interesting phone message left by a patient who was a health-care systems lawyer. He had phoned an insurance company to inquire into buying long-term-care insurance, and was given a memory test by the person at the other end of the line. Apparently, he didn't remember a satisfactory number of words from the list he had been administered, and the insurance company told him that he was at risk for Mild Cognitive Impairment and denied him insurance on these grounds. He had read about me in the newspaper and felt I was a clinician who would sympathize with his plight. Though in our conversations my patient was somewhat enraged by the conduct of the insurance company, I reassured him that the phone diagnosis of "pre-MCI" was inconsequential. My own clinical evaluation showed that he was still of above-average intelligence and experiencing some age-related changes that could be expected of people his age. With renewed confidence in his abilities, he continued to volunteer in the community and conduct his life as a normal person rather than as a diseased one, which included staying engaged in several social organizations that he had been a part of.

THE MAINSTREAM MYTH OF AD

Alzheimer's disease is considered to be the most prevalent form of dementia in the world. It is a progressive, degenerative brain disease characterized by the irreversible death of brain cells. This gradual but poorly understood degeneration leads to shrinkage and atrophy in certain regions of the brain, a decrease in certain neurotransmitters, notably acetylcholine, and an alteration of the synaptic connections between cells that enable us to learn and retain memories.

The overall result of these losses is a variable mental decline that affects the ability to remember recent events, learn new things, and multitask. Doctors don't know what causes the process. More severe changes usually begin after age sixty, and then nearly half of people eighty-five or older (the so-called old-old) are affected. According to most epidemiologists, the rates continue to climb in the 100s (centenarians) and 110s (supercentenarians). But as the standard myth goes, this decline is not a normal part of aging, it is a pathological disease.

The effects of the disease are: memory dysfunction, an impaired ability to learn, reason, make judgments, identify objects, communicate, and maintain a sense of self, profound difficulty carrying out daily activities that require planning, organizing, and motor function, agitation, anxiety, depression, hallucinations, wandering, and insomnia. These deficits are said to be correlated with the presence of particular pathological lesions in the brain caused by two largely protein structures: beta-amyloid protein (BAP) plaques and neurofibrillary tangles (NFTs).

PLAQUES AND TANGLES

Plaques and tangles, both noted by the German psychiatrist Alois Alzheimer, form to one degree or another—and perhaps naturally—over the course of brain aging. In AD the major focus of their effects has been on two regions, the cortex and the hippocampus, where they interfere with normal cognitive functioning and contribute to the death of neurons. Their presence is said to distinguish Alzheimer's-type dementia from vascular dementia, which has a more sudden onset and is caused by blood vessel blockages or bleeding that damages the brain, and Lewy body dementia, characterized by fluctuating cognitive deficits, Parkinsonian motor problems, and the presence of

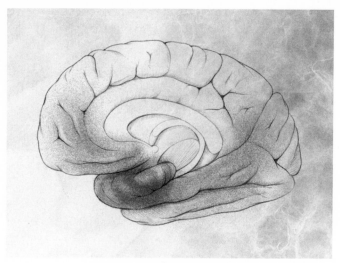

Figure 4A (two images)

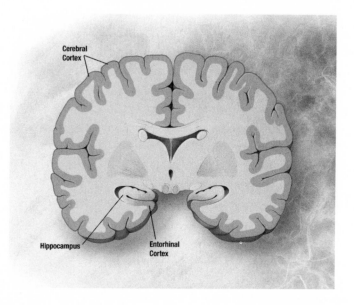

Cerebral
Cortex

Hippocampus

Entorhinal
Cortex

Figure 4. Alzheimer's Brain Changes.   Figures 4A and 4B represent two stages of brain aging. Both figures include two images of the brain as seen in two different views. On the top in both 4A and 4B is a view of the left half (or hemisphere) of the brain viewed from the middle. The reader can imagine that a knife has been used to split the left and right halves of the brain down the middle from front to back. The areas that are shaded in show parts of the brain where pathologists find a high concentration of the two major pathological features of Alzheimer's (plaques that are abnormal nerve cell process surrounding a core of amyloid and neurofibrillary tangles found inside nerve cell bodies). The bottom views in both A and B show the brain as if cuts are made vertically from ear to ear. These sections show the shrinkage of brain tissues in various affected regions. This

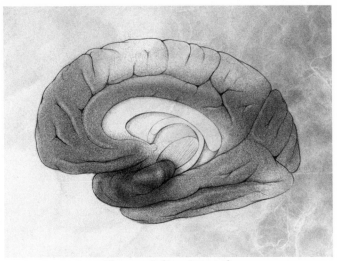

Figure 4B (two images)

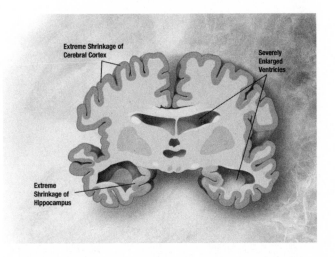

so-called brain atrophy is visible as tissue loss in the folds (called gyri) on the outside of the brain (in the cortex, which means "bark") become more prominent with more space in between the folds. In the top image in 4A (preclinical/normal) there are fewer areas of dense shading, meaning fewer plaques and tangles are found in the brain and their distribution is more limited. This is associated with less shrinkage in the lower panel. This presents normal aging or perhaps preclinical Alzheimer's. In the top image in 4B, representing severe brain aging (or more advanced Alzheimer's changes), the plaques are more widespread and denser in concentration. In the bottom image the atrophy has become more severe (more shrinkage and space between the folds in the cortex). (Courtesy of the National Institute on Aging, *Alzheimer's Disease: Unraveling the Mystery*)

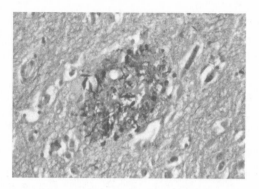

Figure 5. Beta-Amyloid Protein (BAP) Plaque.   BAPs, one of the neuropathological features of Alzheimer's, are composed of a core of beta-amyloid protein surrounded by degenerating nerve cell processes. (Courtesy of the National Institute on Aging, *Alzheimer's Disease: Unraveling the Mystery*)

spherical protein deposits in nerve cells. Plaques and tangles don't show up on routine neuroimaging scans, leaving only two ways to detect their presence: by autopsying the brain after a patient has died or by performing a

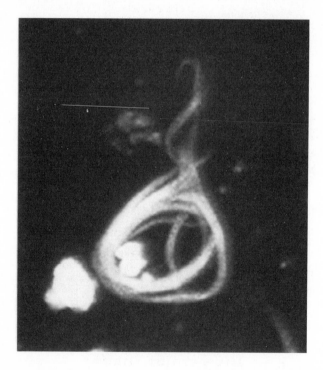

Figure 6. Neurofibrillary Tangle.   Neurofibrillary tangles, which along with BAPs are diagnostic features of Alzheimer's, are composed of abnormal structural proteins inside the nerve cell. (Courtesy of the National Institute on Aging, *Alzheimer's Disease: Unraveling the Mystery*)

biopsy, a diagnostic sampling of brain disease, while the patient is still alive. For obvious safety reasons, and since it rarely leads to any therapeutic intervention, the latter procedure is rarely performed.

A STORY FROM MY PRACTICE

I rarely recommend brain biopsies in my practice. There is one memory that lingers with me of a young man in his twenties who developed cerebral amyloidoma, which is a rare condition in which a form of amyloid protein builds up in the brain like a tumor and damages brain tissue, most likely because it slowly compresses it against the skull. We did a brain biopsy of my young patient to determine his rare condition and thankfully it went safely. We are befuddled by the role of amyloid in the brain. Some think it is the main perpetrator of Alzheimer's disease, while others, including my friend and distinguished colleague George Perry, believe that amyloid buildup may signal other processes, perhaps even a self-repair process in the brain.

Although plaques and tangles are the conventionally accepted perpetrators of Alzheimer's, their respective roles remain controversial and there is a question of whether there is enough evidence to implicate them as causal agents in AD. Scientists are divided on which protein is more to blame. A segment of scientists, referred to as BAPtists, believe that BAP plaques initiate the cell death seen in AD, while a smaller number of scientists, called TAUists, believe that the tau protein tangles are responsible.

There are several other pathological hallmarks of AD, such as Hirano bodies (cytoplasmic protein aggregates that affect the structure of nerve cells) and granulovacuolar degeneration (a failure of cells in the hippocampus characterized by the presence of small granules), which receive almost no funding for study because of the fixation on plaques and tangles.

THE BAPTIST THEORY

Embedded in each neuronal cell membrane is a naturally occurring compound called amyloid precursor protein (APP) that helps neurons grow and survive in ways that science does not yet fully understand. It is believed that APP facilitates communication between cells. In a healthy brain, APP, which is composed of about seven hundred protein building blocks called amino acids, is cleaved and released from the cell membrane by enzymes called secretases. Different types of secretases can act on different portions of the APP, creating peptides that differ in length. Peptides are small proteins composed of amino acids.

If the enzyme alpha-secretase is active, the APP is cleaved in the middle and forms apparently harmless protein fragments. But if the APP is cut by enzymes called beta- and gamma-secretases, the BAP peptide fragment is formed.

This differential pattern of cleavage is important because the amyloid cascade hypothesis holds that this BAP fragment, formed by forty-two amino acids, is toxic to the brain. According to this theory, when the BAP fragment is deposited among neurons, it releases reactive molecules that alter neuronal chemistry, compromise the structure and nutrient transport system of neurons, and may precipitate the formation of tau tangles that lead to cell death and the gradual development of dementia. Lab studies have shown that BAP can kill neurons in Petri dishes and affect connections between neurons in mice models.

While it might seem logical to try to prevent the beta- and gamma-secretases from being present in the brain, the potential of the secretases as therapeutic targets for AD is dampened by the fact that enzymes such as gamma-secretase are involved in various processes throughout the body, including the differentiation of stem cells in bone marrow that develop into red blood cells and lymphocytes. Scientists have tried inhibiting gamma-secretase in mice, but some trials have resulted in toxic effects. Nevertheless, several companies are currently working with gamma-secretase inhibitors in early human trials.

Perhaps the strongest evidence for the amyloid cascade hypothesis came from studies in the 1990s that looked at families who were at especially high risk of getting Alzheimer's. These landmark studies[4] found rare genetic mutations on chromosome 21, which contains the gene encoding for APP production. Mutations on chromosome 21 affect APP production and increase the formation of beta-amyloid protein filaments in the brain that are highly prone to forming the insoluble deposits that supposedly destroy neurons. If one copy of this "faulty" gene is transmitted from parent to child it creates genetic "inevitability"; that is, an

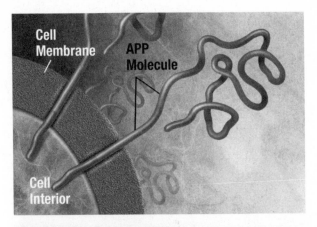

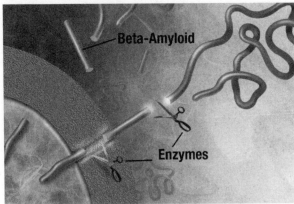

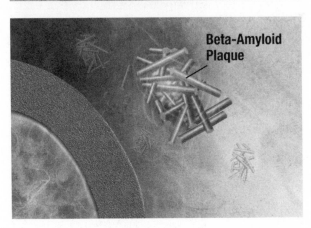

Figure 7. Amyloid Precursor Protein Processing. APP being cut by beta- and gamma-secretase to form a senile plaque shown in a sequence, from top to bottom. (Courtesy of the National Institute on Aging, *Alzheimer's Disease: Unraveling the Mystery*)

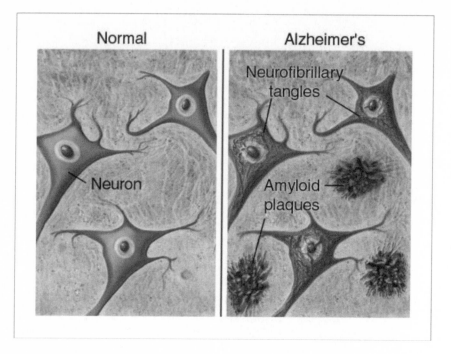

Figure 8. Microscopic View of Alzheimer's.   Comparing a normal brain with a brain affected by plaques and tangles. (Courtesy of the National Institute on Aging, *Alzheimer's Disease: Unraveling the Mystery*)

individual who inherits it will inevitably develop AD symptoms if he or she lives long enough.

Other such "inevitable" mutations have been found on chromosomes 1 and 14, which, like the problems on chromosome 21, cause a strong genetic form of Alzheimer's disease that has a 50 percent probability of being inherited from a parent. These genetic mutations affect molecules called

DIMERS

Most recently scientists have been focusing on so-called dimers and other multiple linked manifestations of the beta-amyloid protein that form in the initial stages before plaque aggregation. *Dimerization* refers to these initial stages in the aggregation, which precede the larger formation of senile plaques. Researchers wonder if in fact these smaller, earlier dimer associations of BAP are the toxic forms, and if plaques are actually sinks that suck up the bad forms and try to prevent the toxic damage of the most soluble forms. In the background, of course, is the question of whether amyloid is toxic to the brain or whether it represents a neural repair mechanism.

presenilins that are related to the presence of gamma-secretase, which affects APP processing and seems to be associated with the formation of the toxic 42-amino acid form of the BAP. Some of these autosomal dominant forms can be diagnosed by finding specific mutations on the aforementioned chromosomes that run in families; and in fact, individuals in these rare families can undergo a blood test and be told whether they're carrying the gene. But this can't be done in every case, since not every case of early-onset Alzheimer's is due to these mutations.

These autosomal mutations on chromosomes 1, 14, and 21 are very rare, affecting perhaps a few thousand families worldwide. But there is a second category of genetic risk factors that have probable risk with regard to the more common late-onset sporadic forms of AD that we see in people age sixty or older.

Autosomal dominant gene mutations on chromosomes 1, 14, and 21 that cause early-onset AD are rare. Susceptibility gene risk factors for late-onset AD have been mapped onto chromosome 19. Thus, there are two basic inherited genetic forms that affect AD risk.

Researchers have found that people carrying a certain variant of a gene mapped to chromosome 19 that controls production of *Apolipoprotein E (ApoE)*—a protein that normally helps transport cholesterol—have an elevated risk of developing Alzheimer's later in life. There are three gene variants—also known as alleles—for ApoE: E2, E3, and E4. Because every child inherits two genes, one from each parent, there are six combinations of alleles:

E2/E2
E3/E3

E4/E4
E2/E3
E2/E4
E3/E4

Combinations containing E4 are associated with a greater probability of AD later in life, with two copies conferring the highest risk. These risk factors will be explored in Chapter 6.

IS IT IN YOUR GENES?

If you elect to undergo genetic testing for AD (although it is not recommended except in a research study), it is imperative to remember that the presence of *ApoE-4 increases susceptibility to Alzheimer's but does not cause the disease by itself. In other words, these are not inevitability genes; they are only susceptibility genes and may increase risk.* In contemporary culture, genes have been accorded a causal power that far exceeds the actual evidence. After all, genes produce other proteins and influence the expression of other genes, but they do this in the complex microenvironment of the cell and macroenvironment of the body in nature. As you will read in Part Three of this book, the occurrence of AD must be explained in a more complex, ecological way.

PROBLEMS WITH THE AMYLOID CASCADE HYPOTHESIS

That is the story as the BAPtists tell it. There are, however, some fundamental problems with the amyloid cascade hypothesis:

1. Scientists still don't understand exactly how beta-amyloid kills neurons. The actual toxicity of the various forms of amyloid has been inconsistently demonstrated and some researchers, including several of my colleagues in Cleveland and elsewhere, believe that amyloid deposition is a secondary phenomenon perhaps even representing

the brain's attempt to launch repair mechanisms in the event of brain injury and compensate for impaired structure or function.[5] George Perry and his colleagues have suggested that amyloid could be an adaptive repair mechanism in the same way that elevated levels of hemoglobin (which is normally toxic when highly concentrated) in the bloodstream are adaptive for human beings at high altitudes.[6] Although controversial, a protective function for amyloid is supported by some literature and also explains why many aged individuals, despite the presence of high numbers of BAP, show little or no cognitive decline. Those who challenge the amyloid cascade hypothesis charge that current therapeutic efforts targeted toward lowering amyloid production or removal of deposited amyloid will only serve to exacerbate the disease process since it may be eliminating a protective agent.[7]

2. Researchers are unsure whether amyloid plaques are responsible for the degeneration of neurons or merely markers or "sears" of where neuronal death has already occurred—essentially, it's a "chicken or egg" problem. As mentioned above, we do not know which form of BAP is toxic in the human brain or even for sure if it is the primary toxin.

3. BAP accumulates in all brains as they age. The process may even start in persons as young as twenty. It would be unnatural for an aging person not to have BAP in their brain, and, in fact, clinical-pathological studies of normal aging individuals demonstrate that nearly one-third of clinically normal people have sufficient levels of amyloid plaques in their brains to warrant an AD diagnosis had they been clinically demented.[8] Thus, to establish a critical threshold of when BAP accumulation becomes a disease is a challenge.

4. There is no consistently strong correlation between plaques and the cognitive impairment of Alzheimer's found across all studies. Variable numbers of plaques (and tangles) are in fact found in the brains of individuals with AD, but these pathological features also appear in normally aged persons who are not diagnosed with any cognitive dysfunction during their lives. As I mentioned, it is sometimes the case that individuals whose brains exhibit high levels of plaques, often exceeding the criteria for AD, will test as highly on cognitive performance as individuals with low BAP count. Conversely, persons

with diagnosed AD are occasionally found to have less of a concentration of plaques on their brains than persons who presented no Alzheimer's symptoms in their later life. The possible explanation: Some people's brains are simply more resilient to plaques than others. *Thus, the existence of BAP in a brain does not necessarily mean that a person will exhibit AD in their life.*

You can see that the jury is still out on plaques. In spite of this uncertainty, considerable effort is being spent on developing drugs that would inhibit the action of the beta- and gamma-secretases in an effort to prevent the formation of the allegedly toxic 42-amino acid BAP fragment. Once again, I must emphasize that amyloid precursor protein and some of its constituents play a role in normal function of the brain. It is not clear that altering its metabolism will necessarily benefit patients; and such actions could even cause harm.

THE TAUIST STORY

TAUists think they have a better theory to explain Alzheimer's disease, and their story goes like this. Some tangles form from intercellular tau proteins as part of the process of aging, but others may be the result of a disease process. Normally, the tau protein is thought to have at least two roles in the human nervous system. The protein supports a neuron's structure like a microscopic trellis, and regulates nutrient transport much like an intercellular pipeline. With Alzheimer's disease, scientists conjecture that the tau protein undergoes a chemical change and becomes stickier due to a process of phosphoryllation (whereby small compounds called phosphates are added to the chemical structure of tau, possibly altering its structure).

Perhaps in association with this alteration in the phosphate metabolism, the tau proteins pair up and bind to each other, forming densely twisted coils that merge into larger intracellular tangles that, in turn, clog the neuronal axons and dendrites, the branching parts of neurons that link up with other brain cells and allow for basic communication. The stable support and nutrition transport system inside neurons collapses and this leads to miscommunication between neurons, incapacitated nutrient flow, and eventual cell death from malnutrition. TAUists claim that the intracellular BAP plaques are a secondary by-product of tau tangle formation rather than the other way around.

THE TRUTH ABOUT PLAQUES AND TANGLES

Arguments continue as to whether the BAP found *around* the brain's neurons or the neurofibrillary tangles found *inside* the brain's neurons are more important in the cognitive dysfunction of AD. Even though there remains a weak correlation between amyloid plaques and cognitive dysfunction, and no definitive proof to distinguish amyloid as the lone perpetrator of Alzheimer's disease, the BAPtists have dominated the field for the past decade, monopolizing funding and blocking research into other fruitful areas of biological and psychosocial research, including quality of life, caregiving, and early preventive medicine. In their attempts to cure Alzheimer's, the BAPtists are gunning, in part, for Nobel Prizes and personal wealth. If they succeed (which I doubt) they will deserve our gratitude; but in the meantime, much fame and fortune has been generated on the basis of hype and hope rather than on product and outcome.

MOVING PAST PLAQUES AND TANGLES

It is likely that Alzheimer's is not the result of a lone biological factor, or even a tandem of microscopic perpetrators. Remember, few credible scientists I know believe in the myth that Alzheimer's is a singular disease, process, or condition, and many believe as I do that Alzheimer's is a blanket label that subsumes many of the processes of normal brain aging. Brain aging is caused by a confluence of genetic, environmental, and behavioral factors—hence people's trajectory along the brain-aging continuum varies immensely.

A landmark longitudinal investigation of Alzheimer's disease and aging, called the Nun Study, which was the cover story of *Time* in May 2001, reinforced how little we know about the toxicity of plaques and tangles in AD. The study was conducted on 678 American members of the School of Sisters of Notre Dame religious order. For decades, researchers traced the cognitive development and degeneration of these cloistered women, scrutinizing everything from their writings as twenty-year-olds to their memory retention in old age to their postmortem brains. These postmortem exams were especially revealing, as the Nun Study provided significant evidence that elderly persons may still function normally with relatively high concentrations of plaques and tangles on their brains, while those with the cognitive and behavioral symptoms of

Alzheimer's disease may often be found to have a relatively smaller plaque concentration.

> ### MORE ON PLAQUES AND TANGLES
>
> In *This Room Is Yours,* the author, Michael Stein, provides a helpful way of viewing the plaques and tangles of AD. He writes: "Both people with Alzheimer's diagnoses and the 'normal' elderly would have plaques and tangles if we lined up pieces of their frontal lobes on [a] coffee table; if these tangles were quantified there would be a clear overlap among the two groups."[9]

No easy correlation exists between the presence of these two antagonists and Alzheimer's disease. There is no easy answer to what causes the dementia in AD; no one or two assailants we can attack with biological therapies. In the absence of causal clarity, multiple competing theories of causation have emerged.

THE ANTIOXIDANT HYPOTHESIS

The antioxidant hypothesis of Alzheimer's disease is a relatively old one that has resurfaced in different ways over the years to explain both AD and normal aging. The premise of the theory is that free radicals—atoms or groups of atoms that have at least one unpaired electron and are therefore weakly bonded, unstable, and highly reactive—accumulate in the brain, damaging nerve cells and resulting in loss of cell function, which could contribute to AD. These molecules are produced in the body by natural biological processes, and can be accelerated by external agents such as infections, tobacco smoke, toxins, herbicides, radiation from the sun, or pollutants. Free radicals can damage proteins by altering their chemical structure and DNA and potentially causing mutations.

Essentially, when molecules split as a result of bodily metabolism—a natural process by which chemicals in our body are created and destroyed—free radicals are born and react quickly with other nearby compounds to try to regain stability. These free radicals effectively "steal" electrons from other molecules, setting off a cascade of disruptions that can detrimentally affect living cells, including neurons. Normally the body can stabilize free radicals on its own, but if antioxidants are unavailable in one's diet or if free radical production becomes excessive, damage can occur, and can be especially profound on proteins, lipids, and nucleic acids (RNA and DNA). Cells possess DNA-repair enzymes that replace nucleotide (abbreviated by A, C, T, G) pairs, but it becomes an increasingly uphill battle as we age. The damage that free radicals inflict on our microscopic building blocks compromises cell function, organ function, and potentially the functioning of major body systems. In humans, it is thought that this free-radical damage can accelerate the progression of cancer, cardiovascular disease, and age-related degenerative diseases like AD. Though this is likely true, the antioxidant theory can only partially account for the widespread multi-system damage caused in so-called AD.

A variety of antioxidant drugs are thought to slow down the damage associated with free radicals. However, actual clinical trials of antioxidants have been disappointing.

One such product, vitamin E, has been widely recommended by experts to slow progression of AD and aging in general, although this approach is now falling out of favor. Recent studies have failed to confirm initial impressions that vitamin E may be helpful in slowing the progression of memory problems.[10] In fact, in 2005, researchers at Johns Hopkins reported that doses of vitamin E in excess of 400 milligrams have serious risks, and may be associated with a higher overall risk of mortality.[11]

Other experts recommend eating antioxidant-rich diets full of fruits and vegetables, since it is theorized that such antioxidants as vitamins E and C and selenium may have the capacity to neutralize free radicals by donating their electrons to help with stability. An abundance of antioxidants, it is held, may preempt the chain reaction of damage to living cells in the body.

These theories withstanding, the long-term effects of antioxidants have not been proven.

THE INFLAMMATORY HYPOTHESIS

In recent years, the inflammatory hypothesis has achieved some prominence in the AD community, because inflammatory molecules are often associated with senile plaques. According to the hypothesis, AD arises as a consequence of brain inflammation, which creates abnormal metabolites—small molecular products of metabolic processes—from normal brain molecules. The inflammation process that creates these metabolites can be triggered by numerous stimuli, including infections or traumatic head injuries that predate the onset of Alzheimer's disease by a significant amount of time— perhaps even years or decades. These abnormal metabolites, along with such normal reactive immune system proteins as cytokines, are produced by tissue inflammation and may course through the brain, modifying beta-amyloid proteins and causing them to form into the aforementioned insoluble beta-amyloid plaques.[12]

WATCH YOUR HEAD

Recent studies have shown that head injury elevates the associated risk of those carrying the ApoE-4 susceptibility gene. Richard Mayeux and colleagues[13] found a two-fold risk for dementia when ApoE-4 was present without a head injury, but a ten-fold increase from the combination of ApoE-4 and a head injury.

Because beta-amyloid proteins and plaques are considered to be associated with inflammation in AD, the inflammatory hypothesis has received some credence. Some see inflammation as the lead event to beta-amyloid protein plaque production, while those in the BAPtist camp see inflammation as a secondary event and defend their protein as the hallmark of AD. Still others see the inflammatory markers simply as innocent bystanders, having no bearing on cognitive dysfunction.

Once again, initial studies of people with memory problems provided evidence that such nonsteroidal anti-inflammatory drugs (NSAIDs) as ibuprofen, naproxen, and indomethacin might be helpful for brain health, but these early studies were not replicated. Taking these drugs can cause serious side effects like bleeding in the gastrointestinal system.

THE EXCITATORY CELL DEATH HYPOTHESIS

Other studies have implicated the mechanism of excitatory cell death (ECD) in AD. In the ECD theory, neurons are thought to die through excess stimulation by excitatory amino acid neurotransmitters. In models produced in animals, where an excess amount of a normally present neurotransmitter like glutamate is administered, neurons tend to die. Because glutamate and other excitatory neurotransmitters normally cause the nerve cells to fire electrically, it is believed that, in excess, they cause neurons to fire (excite) themselves to death.

Although it is fairly easy to demonstrate this destructive process in a variety of experimental circumstances, for example nerve cells isolated in a dish, no one is sure that this excitatory damage actually occurs in any natural disease process.

THE INFECTIOUS DISEASE HYPOTHESIS

Occasionally, scientists have claimed to have established evidence of viral and other infections in the brains of patients with Alzheimer's. These so-called slow viruses known as prions are made of proteins rather than DNA or RNA, as are most viruses, and cause such conditions as Creutzfeldt-Jakob disease, kuru, scrapie, and the infamous mad cow disease (bovine spongiform encephalopathy).

Prions were discovered by the American scientist Stanley Prusiner in the 1980s and have been found to cause spongiform encephalopathies—brain pathology marked by small holes in brain tissue. In some cases, they have been found to leave protein aggregates in the form of amyloid deposits in their wake, similar but not identical to those found in Alzheimer's disease. Early attempts to transmit AD through inoculation of diseased human tissue into animal brains were not replicated. Certain herpes viruses and other infectious diseases can cause dementia, but they are not consistently related to Alzheimer's. Further, evidence that infectious agents have been present in a person's brain does not necessarily mean that they are the agents causing the dementia. Most of the claims that infectious agents are producing AD are never replicated in follow-up studies by different scientists.

THE VASCULAR HYPOTHESIS

Many parallels have been drawn between similar causative mechanisms in AD and vascular dementia by focusing on pathology in blood vessels. It has long been known that strokes, sudden blockage or rupture of a blood vessel supplying a part of the brain, can lead to the death of brain tissue, which causes cognitive impairment. Strokes that damage the left hemisphere of the brain can cause language impairment (*aphasia*), while strokes on the right can cause visual-spatial problems—for example, poor drawing skills, getting lost, or having difficulty tying shoes. Strategic single small infarcts, or clots, in critical regions of the brain or multiple small blood vessel blockages can cause dementia by reducing the brain's oxygen supply and disrupting nerve cell circuits involved in decision making, memory, and verbal skills.

Before plaques and tangles were dragged out as the main suspects in AD, it was thought that stroke-related dementias were the most common causes of cognitive impairment. Many patients seem to have mixed dementia: a cluster of vascular and degenerative processes that, considered together, complicate a straight AD diagnosis.

THE ALZHEIMER'S-DIABETES HYPOTHESIS

In the summer of 2006, the Tenth International Conference on Alzheimer's Disease and Related Disorders was held in Madrid, Spain. At the conference the buzz was that there was a clear link between diabetes and dementia. Diabetes had been known for some time to be a risk factor for vascular diseases like heart attack and stroke. Disturbances in glucose metabolism had been reported in Alzheimer's disease decades ago, with scientists theorizing that either the brain of a diabetic person lacks sufficient glucose to function properly or excess sugar in a diabetic person's bloodstream does vascular damage that affects blood flow to neurons.

In Madrid, evidence was presented to suggest that antidiabetic drugs could be used as a treatment for AD. Epidemiological studies suggested that people with Alzheimer's had co-occurring diabetes more than those who did not, while other studies showed that people with high blood pressure and prediabetes tended to score poorly on cognitive tests. Further, small pilot randomized controlled studies reported that drugs used to treat diabetes led to some improvements in patients. As is quite common in these small clinical studies, the results were overinterpreted. Undoubtedly, there is a scientific basis to some of the interrelationships between glucose metabolism and dementia, but I worry that the Alzheimer's-diabetes link is another example of cure mongering—the latest AD story du jour.

> ### ADDING IT ALL UP
>
> Some claim that the emergence of these varying perspectives on the causes of Alzheimer's disease represents progress. To me, it represents more confusion. Perhaps some clarity can be gained by recognizing that aging has many manifestations and hence that the brain aging we now call Alzheimer's disease has multiple biological causes and factors as well.

THE AD DIAGNOSIS: A CLINICAL QUANDARY

What most people don't know is that, despite the certitude displayed by those who study and treat Alzheimer's disease and spread the simplistic story to the public, the criteria that doctors use to diagnose patients with AD stipulate that a definitive diagnosis can only be made in postmortem examination. Even the postmortem examination is problematic, because, as emphasized earlier, there is no direct correlation involving BAP and NFT. Even pathologists must ask the clinician whether the patient was demented or not in their life in order to consider a diagnosis of Alzheimer's in death.

Another reason for the lack of diagnostic certainty in AD is that many people can be seen to have an overlap of vascular problems, Lewy bodies, and plaques and tangles—all of these pathologies arise in all of our brains as we age. More baffling yet is that the appearance of these pathologies doesn't always correlate with behavioral symptoms. In other words, as was the case in the Nun Study, people may be found upon autopsy to have a high concentration of pathological features on their brains, but may have presented fewer symptoms of dementia than another patient who was found to have lower concentrations of pathological features on their brain.

We treat Alzheimer's disease as if it was as real as the plague, and yet, even the top experts in the field can't precisely diagnose it. The disease is a moving target, a chimera. As one of the textbooks in the field, *Psychiatry in the Elderly,* puts it: "The pathology of [AD] defies precise definition at present. This is because its individual components all occur to some extent in normal aging."[14]

This means that any diagnosis given during your or a loved one's life can only be probable—the best judgment of neurologists like me. There is never any point at which you or a loved one becomes an Alzheimer's victim.

No one common set of symptoms or quantifiable pathological characteristics can establish a human being as having Alzheimer's disease.

In AD, each individual case is different. In fact, many of us in the AD field have a saying that goes "Once you've seen one patient with Alzheimer's, you've seen one patient with Alzheimer's." There is no one biological marker in Alzheimer's patients that is consistent from person to person. Every individual with presumed AD has a brain that moves along the continuum of brain aging in a unique way.

As you can see, there are no clear boundaries delineating normal aging from Alzheimer's disease or the other dementias; Ralph Waldo Emerson may have put it best when he observed that "all diseases run into one: old age." Alzheimer's is not so much a monster that terrorizes the neurons in our brains as it is a conceptual phantom lurking in the shadows of our psyche.

There is no cure for the common birthday.
—JOHN GLENN

A DISEASE OF EXCLUSION

If you or a loved one is diagnosed with Alzheimer's disease, you need to consider how exactly the doctor has made the diagnosis, and whether the diagnosis is sound.

From a conceptual standpoint, it's helpful to compare AD to an infectious disease like HIV/AIDS. Though both diseases inspire a nearly universal fear in all of us, HIV/AIDS has a clear-cut etiology (origin). Blood tests can be used to identify the virus and its antibodies and establish definitively whether one is a carrier of the disease or not. Alzheimer's, which we already know is a probable diagnosis, even upon autopsy, is not so simple to identify. Today clinicians who assess older persons with cognitive problems assess the AD label as a diagnosis of exclusion, which means that a diagnosis of AD can only be made if other causes such as the following can be ruled out:

Hypothyroidism and other metabolic causes
Vascular problems like stroke
Vitamin deficiencies, including B_{12}
Hypercalcemia

Normal pressure hydrocephalus
Psychiatric difficulties like depression and schizophrenia
Head trauma
Structural brain lesions—brain tumors, injuries, or blood clots
Other degenerative conditions like Parkinson's disease
Malingering and factitious disorder
Dehydration and other causes of delirium
Brain infections like HIV, encephalitis, meningitis, syphilis
Chronic effects of various substances, including alcohol and other
   medications

The truth is we can only make a "probable" diagnosis of AD once we have eliminated all other causes. We cannot even make a definite diagnosis of Alzheimer's if we examine brain tissue.

As well as being a diagnosis of exclusion, AD is a label that excludes by branding patients whose brains are aging with a stigmatizing disease, and introduces anguish, fear, and slow resignation into people's lives. *Every time the diagnosis of Alzheimer's is made, we must remember that it can be as socially destructive as it is scientifically uncertain.*

CHAPTER THREE

THE TROUBLING LEGACY OF DR. ALOIS ALZHEIMER AND AUGUSTE D.

> *Concepts, like individuals, have their histories and are just as incapable of withstanding the ravages of time as are individuals.*
>
> —SØREN KIERKEGAARD

In December 1995, my friend Konrad Maurer, a professor of psychiatry at the University of Frankfurt, and two of his colleagues made the discovery of a lifetime. Scouring through the bowels of the Johann Wolfgang Goethe Frankfurt University Hospital, Konrad and his colleagues happened upon a cardboard box full of dusty old papers and portfolios—patient records dating back to the mid-twentieth century. Konrad's colleague pulled out a handful of blue-colored cardboard files from the box. Noticing that one set was significantly older and more worn than the others, he scrutinized it more closely, and then spun to his colleagues and shouted, "This is Auguste D.!"[1]

Konrad and his colleagues reported feeling like young boys who had just unearthed a buried treasure, for this, they believed—with some justification—was one of twentieth-century medicine's landmark historical document finds: Dr. Alois Alzheimer's original folio of case materials and handwritten records of his most famed patient, Auguste Deter. Frau Deter, or "Auguste D." as she is best known to posterity, was the wife of a railway clerk whose early-onset dementia at age fifty-one became the basis for the framework of Alzheimer's disease.

The materials found by Konrad and his colleagues—a total of thirty-two sheets with the patient's admission report, an attestation, and three versions of the case history in Latin and German[2]—illuminated the day-to-day clinical and pathological work performed by Dr. Alzheimer during his milestone case from 1901 to 1906 and revealed the doctor to be a most circumspect clinician who devoted himself to his patients with empathy and skill, while keeping precise accounts of each case. The transcripts of the interviews with Auguste D. are difficult to interpret, as they represent the doctor's clinical notes. At times he appears empathetic, and at other times somewhat aggressive in questioning Auguste D. about her name, her husband's name, and her address. Although the materials illuminated Dr. Alzheimer's personal idiosyncrasies as a clinician, they did not create a clear picture of the disease named after him. In fact, his writings revealed that Alzheimer himself was not sure how Auguste D. fit into the continuum of senility and dementia, and showed that basic clinical and pathological features observed in Auguste D. were seen to be just as confusing to Alzheimer and his colleagues in 1906 as they are to us a century later.

The severe memory loss, cognitive impairment, aphasia (a loss of the ability to produce words or comprehend language), apraxia (a loss in the ability to perform skilled movements), delusions, and hallucinations observed in Auguste D., as well as the neuronal loss, high plaque and tangle count, and arteriosclerotic changes discovered in her brain upon postmortem, were virtually identical to the clinical symptoms, pathological hallmarks, and disease progression of senile dementia—the type of dementia known to afflict persons in their later years.

> Dr. Alzheimer could see amyloid at the core of senile plaques through his microscope but did not know it was a protein. Even though we now use high-tech devices called PET scans to image amyloid in living patients, we still do not know how it is involved in normal functions and if and how it can harm the brain.

Maurer's discovery in 1995 has helped us come to realize the troubling path from Auguste D.'s condition to what we now call Alzheimer's disease.

PORTRAIT OF A YOUNG DOCTOR

Dr. Alois Alzheimer was a stout and powerfully built man, born June 4, 1864, in Marktbreit am Main, a village in lower Franconia in the southern Bavaria region of Germany. In 1998 I had an opportunity to visit his family house, which has been converted into a small conference center where we held our own conference exploring concepts of Alzheimer's disease. During his lifetime, Dr. Alzheimer was known as a pioneering researcher, a colorful character in medical school classrooms, and a genial family man. The avuncular Alzheimer wore pince-nez spectacles and was rarely seen without a cigar in his mouth.

In the summer of 1886, the twenty-two-year-old graduated from medical school after studying at three different universities. During his studies, he developed a lifelong passion for histology—the microscopic study of the structure of human tissues—and set the foundation for his unprecedented observations in the fields of epilepsy, brain tumors, Huntington's disease, alcoholic delirium, syphilis (a common cause of dementia at the time), and what became known as Alzheimer's disease.

At the age of twenty-four, he was hired as an asylum officer at the Stadtische Irrenstalt Mental Asylum in Frankfurt. The clinic was a sprawling facility, a thirty-seven-acre complex of splendidly built pavilions and covered walkways and surrounded by parks, esplanades, and gardens. It was subdivided into units for the paralytic, the imbecilic, the raving, and the epileptic. Here he commenced his practical education in psychiatry and devoted himself to his main interest, neuropathology.[3]

It was also where he first encountered Auguste D., the patient who would come to be known as the first "Alzheimer's" patient in the world.

MEETING AUGUSTE D.

According to Konrad Maurer's reconstruction of the events, on November 26, 1901, Alzheimer came across a file that his assistant Dr. Paul Nitsche had marked "Auguste D." Alzheimer browsed the file once, read it over more carefully a second time, and soon became so engrossed that he could not put it down. This patient presented an anomaly like he had never seen.

According to Auguste D.'s husband, the couple had been harmoniously married since 1873. She had borne one daughter, suffered no miscarriages, and was otherwise described as hardworking and orderly. At most she was somewhat excitable and nervous but otherwise "rather amicable." She had no disease history, drank no alcohol, and did not take drugs. The husband reported that his wife began showing signs of confusion in March 1901, when she made groundless accusations that her husband was out walking with a female neighbor. From then on, she harbored an implacable jealousy of her husband and a loathing for the neighbor.

The husband noted a gradual decline in his wife's short- and long-term memory. She became restive and absentminded, making obvious mistakes in food preparation, neglecting her housework, stashing all sorts of small objects in nooks and crannies around the apartment, and wandering aimlessly from room to room with a vacant stare. She spoke frequently of death and began to insist that a courier who often came into the house had the intention of harming her. After eight months of managing and enduring his wife's rapid decline, Auguste D.'s husband admitted her into Alzheimer's institution. On the admittance notice, the family doctor had written:

> Mrs. Auguste D., wife of the railway clerk Mr. Carl D., Morfelder Land-strasse, has been suffering for a long time from weakness of memory, persecution mania, sleeplessness, restlessness. She is unable to perform any physical or mental work. Her condition (chronic brain paresis) needs treatment from the local mental institution.[4]

Something about the peculiarities of Auguste D.'s case captivated Alzheimer, and the doctor wanted to meet the patient for himself. And so, on this November morning, he came face-to-face with Auguste D.

Despite her manifold symptoms, the fifty-one-year-old patient, a slight woman with long black hair and wizened skin, had an affable demeanor. She could write her full name if told each individual word but had trouble putting sentences together and showed signs of verbal perseveration, a condition in which one repeats words or phrases. Constantly fearful of those around her, Auguste D. hoarded her possessions under her hospital bed and avoided others except on rare occasions when she would walk around the asylum groping the faces of fellow patients. She regarded Dr. Alzheimer with suspicion, often growing lachrymose and refusing, or being unable, to cooperate when the doctor posed his questions.

TRACKING THE CASE

As the months went by, the case of Auguste D. stayed with Dr. Alzheimer. Years before, he had observed cases of age-induced feeble-mindedness in much older patients, but never in someone as young as Auguste D. He suspected that senile dementia could be brought on by the thickening of the blood vessels of the brain—a condition called atheriosclerosis—and published an article, "Dementia Senilis and Brain Disease Based on Atheromatous Vessel Disease," in the *Monthly Journal of Psychiatry,* 1898.

Nearly a year into Auguste D.'s illness, Dr. Alzheimer reviewed her hospital admission sheet, which would remain hidden away for the next ninety years. Next to the heading of "Causes of Illness" he put "arteriosclerosis," and in the form of illness section he wrote "arteriosclerotic brain atrophy," but rather tellingly flagged the entry with a question mark.

ARTERIOSCLEROSIS

Arteriosclerosis is a chronic disease in which thickening, hardening, and loss of elasticity of the arterial walls result in impaired blood circulation. It develops with aging, and is associated with hypertension, diabetes, hyperlipidemia, and other conditions.

Considering the terror spawned by the condition that now bears Alzheimer's name, it is ironic that the doctor's final note on Auguste D.'s sheet, under the heading of "Form of Illness," was "simple mental disorder."

Still, Alzheimer recognized that the case could prove to be of scientific importance because of Auguste D.'s young age. At fifty-one, she exhibited the behavioral symptoms that one might expect to observe in a dementia patient in their seventh, eighth, or ninth decade. Along with his Italian colleague Gaetano Perusini, Alzheimer evaluated three additional cases in addition to Auguste D. (at death, aged forty-six, sixty, and sixty-five) of presenile dementia.[5] The dilemma for Alzheimer and his colleagues was the same one we face today: Did Auguste D. and others have a specific disease, or were their brains aging and experiencing the symptoms of senility a bit more rapidly than others? This quandary puzzled Alzheimer for the years to come. He arranged for precise documentation of the course of Auguste D.'s illness, instructing the clinic photographer to take a number of pictures of his patient, including the portraits that were later found by Konrad Maurer and his colleagues in the basement of the Frankfurt hospital.

EMIL KRAEPELIN: AN IMPORTANT CRAFTSMAN OF THE AD MYTH

These materials might have been insignificant historical detritus if it hadn't been for Emil Kraepelin, a leading international psychiatrist, and a man whom history might well remember as the real father of Alzheimer's disease. In 1902, Kraepelin offered Alzheimer a chance to join his research team in Heidelberg. Alzheimer already knew the background of the prolific Kraepelin, who was six years Alzheimer's senior and came from Neustrelitz in Mecklenburg. Kraepelin, like Alzheimer, had studied medicine in Würzburg and passed the state exams there. He went on to work at various training sites, including asylums, psychiatric clinics, and outpatient clinics throughout Germany.

At the urgings of his colleagues, Kraepelin had begun publishing his psychiatry textbooks in 1883, and by the twentieth century, these books were known worldwide. Alzheimer eagerly anticipated collaborating with an outstanding researcher and taxonomist like Kraepelin, because Kraepelin shared his belief that mental illness should be predicated on brain pathology rather than Freudian theorizing about the psyche. In addition, he realized that the chances of becoming a university professor would be strengthened by joining forces with such a formidable figure.

Kraepelin's lab featured notable international researchers from Italy, the United States, England, France, Norway, and Switzerland, and offered Alzheimer the chance to immerse himself in his own lab research. Even so, the economic condition of the clinic declined, resulting in deficits and the overcrowding of patients.

AMERICA'S EARLY LINK TO DR. ALZHEIMER

Alzheimer had many pupils visit and work in his laboratory, many of whom became quite famous in their own right. Solomon Fuller was born in Liberia, the grandson of a freed slave. After moving to the United States for his undergraduate work at the University of North Carolina he attended Boston College Medical School and received advanced training in psychiatry and neuropathology. He worked with Kraepelin, Alzheimer, and Franz Nissl from 1904 to 1905 and published the first cases of Alzheimer's disease in English in 1912. Like Alzheimer, he was well known for his careful preparation and analysis of brain tissues, and he was likely helpful to Alzheimer in his analysis of the first cases. Fuller returned to the United States where he eventually became the first African-American professor at Boston University School of Medicine.

In 1903, when Kraepelin was offered the director's position of the Royal Psychiatric Clinic in Munich, he jumped at the offer and asked Alzheimer to join his team.

A month after Alzheimer arrived in Munich, he presented his thesis, entitled "Histological Studies of General Paresis," to the Higher Medical Faculty of the Ludwig-Maximilian University in Munich. Kraepelin offered unequivocal praise of Alzheimer's work, describing the thesis as being "an extraordinary achievement," one showing that "its author is a mature researcher who unquestionably is prepared to join the teaching body of a university."[6]

"ON A PECULIAR, SEVERE DISEASE PROCESS . . ."

In the autumn of 1906, Kraepelin named Alzheimer his chief leading physician, a promotion that had the unfortunate consequence of pulling Alzheimer away from his scientific research. Later that fall, on November 3, Alzheimer delivered his now-famous lecture, "On a Peculiar, Severe Disease Process of the Cerebral Cortex," to the 37th Assembly of Southwest German Alienists (Psychologists) in Tübingen, his college town. Alzheimer stood before nearly ninety of his colleagues and reported on the case of Auguste D. and her progressive cognitive impairment, hallucinations, delusions, marked psychosocial incompetence, and focal symptoms relating to higher cortical dysfunction. Alzheimer interspersed his lecture with wonderfully drawn slides of the amyloid plaques and tangles found in and on the patient's brain in postmortem investigation.

THE STORY OF AMYLOID

Amyloid was first identified by the German professor and physician Dr. R. L. K. Virchow in 1853. Virchow described the reaction of the seemingly abnormal extracellular material with iodine and sulfuric acid, which, at the time, was a marker for starch; and thus, he applied the term *amyloid,* which is derived from the Greek word *amylon,* meaning "starch." Virchow's mislabeling of amyloid as a starch persisted until the 1980s when the American researcher George Glenner identified the molecular structure of amyloid as a protein and proposed its relation to Alzheimer's disease. Despite Virchow's error, his contributions to medicine and public health are formidable. He was one of the first advocates for modern water and sewage systems in the West, which drastically reduced the spread of disease and death. Scholars such as the humanist Harvard physician Paul Farmer also credit Virchow with establishing the field of social medicine, which is predicated on the understanding that disease is never purely biological but also has many contributing social factors.

From what limited records we have of the meeting, it would seem that those on hand were not overly impressed. The minutes of the proceedings reported that the lecture had been "inappropriate for a brief report."[7] No questions were posed following Dr. Alzheimer's presentation since there was no ensuing discussion over his claims. The *Tübingen Chronicle* gave only a brief sentence alluding to Alzheimer's report, reporting: "Dr. Alzheimer from Munich gave an account of a peculiarly severe disease process, which caused a significant shrinkage of the nerve cells within four and a half years."[8]

The tepid response was a setback for Alzheimer, and may have reinforced his questioning of whether the symptoms he observed in Auguste D. constituted a disease separate from senile dementia.

In several months, Alzheimer's lecture in Tübingen appeared, in full, in the *General Journal of Psychiatry and Psycho-Forensic Medicine* under the rubric "Proceedings of Psychiatric Associations." And in early 1907, Alzheimer published a three-page report, "On a Peculiar Disease of the Cerebral Cortex," officially presenting the case of Auguste D.'s presenile dementia to the world.

THE BIRTH OF THE LABEL

In 1910, Emil Kraepelin officially coined the term *Alzheimer's krankheit* ("Alzheimer's disease") when he referred to it for the first time on page 627 of the eighth edition of his authoritative *Psychiatry* textbook. The entry begins with this not-so-illustrious sentence: "The clinical interpretation of Alzheimer's disease is still unclear at the moment." After leading with this disclaimer, Kraepelin continues: "Whereas the anatomic findings suggest that we are dealing with a severe form of senile dementia, the fact that the disease from time to time begins at the end of the patient's forties speaks against it. In such cases at least one would therefore have to assume a presenile dementia, if we are not in fact dealing with a peculiar disease process that is largely independent of age."[9]

Alzheimer felt uncomfortable with the eponymous label. In an article he submitted to the *Zeitschrift fur die Gesamte Neurologie and Psychiatrie* in 1911, he wrote: "The question arises whether these cases of disease, which I have considered as peculiar, still show characteristic features in clinical and histological aspects that distinguish them from senile dementia or whether they must be assigned instead to senile dementia itself."[10]

Alzheimer even alludes to the ambivalence of his boss, writing: "Kraepelin still considers that the position of these cases is unclear." And later he answers the question that he initially posed by concluding that "there is, then, no tenable reason to consider these cases as caused by a specific disease process. They are senile psychoses, atypical forms of senile dementia. Nevertheless, they do assume a certain separate position so that one has to know of their existence."[11]

More and more, a picture emerges of a scientist who was reluctant to see a peculiar form of dementia elevated as a separate disease category, especially in the absence of differentiating biomarkers. Yet Kraepelin had a stake in creating a new disease category. The central question becomes: Why would Emil Kraepelin, a man of strict professional discipline and a thoroughgoing fealty to scientific methodology, reify a disease that he himself deemed "unclear," especially when, as his colleague Alzheimer wrote in 1911, there seemed to be "a variety of intermediate forms between presenile and senile dementia"? Two plausible theories implicate pride, prestige, reputation, and financial pressures as decisive factors that influenced Kraepelin's decision.

SHOWERED WITH PRAISE IN HIS TIME

Ironically, Dr. Alzheimer attained much more fame and notoriety in his lifetime for the bath treatments he developed to soothe patients with manic and paralytic states of excitation than he did for the disease that bears his name. In Germany physicians still prescribe trips to the spa for what ails their patients.

PICK'S LAB: FANNING THE COMPETITIVE FIRES

As the philosopher Thomas Kuhn points out, new scientific theories are often brought about because of factors extrinsic to science: "Conversions occur not despite the fact that scientists are human but because they are."[12] Kraepelin, known as the "pope" and "Linnaeus" of psychiatry, had amassed the respect and reputation that entitled him to name a disease after one of his loyal coworkers. He may have published the AD section in his textbook to establish the fame of one of his junior colleagues, thereby increasing the prestige and dominance of his own school of psychiatry in Munich.[13] Kraepelin's lab, which struggled financially, was in competition with the German Psychiatric Clinic in Prague, Czechoslovakia, run by Arnold Pick, for whom Pick's disease, a progressive disorder of the brain, is named. The two labs were juggernauts in the study of neuropsychiatry and neuropathology, and, as major rivals tend to do, competed over who would be Europe's arbiter of mental psychosis.

In 1907, Pick's coworker Otto Fischer had published interesting findings on the same amyloid brain plaques that Alzheimer had observed in Auguste D., but did not support a separate diagnosis. He preferred the term *presbyophrenic dementia* to describe elderly patients with memory loss, disorientation, and verbal dysfunction. Seen in this light, Kraepelin's creation of Alzheimer's disease established a diagnostic territory over which the Munich lab could reign. Besides elevating Alzheimer's work over Fischer's, the designation of the disease category lent credibility and clout to Kraepelin's lab and created justification for supporting further research into diseases of society's aging citizens.[14]

THE FREUDIAN SCHOOL: DUELING DIAGNOSES

Other historians theorize that the rift between Kraepelin and Sigmund Freud played a role in establishing Alzheimer's disease. In 1900, Freud published *The Interpretation of Dreams,* which captivated not only his colleagues, but also lay readers far and wide. Freud's theory revolutionized the study of neurosis by attributing symptoms of psychiatric diseases to the mysterious workings of the unconscious and suggesting that those neuroses could be treated by bringing unconscious wishes and repressed memories to consciousness through psychoanalytic treatment.

Freudian theory represented direct opposition to Alzheimer's and Kraepelin's organic-based psychiatric views.[15] For them, neurological illnesses had a purely organic basis that could be ascertained by means of scientific inquiry. The Freudian contention that some of the symptoms seen in patients like Auguste D. were caused by the psychic slag left over from traumatic childhood memories seemed an intellectual farce, an aesthetic guessing game in the guise of science. Kraepelin wrote: "What is known so far about this interpretive art makes it appear completely conceivable that psychoanalysis could simply never become common property; it is obviously more art than science. . . . The procedure therefore can never be of general value, at least as long as it has its current goals."[16] In his latest book on Freud, the historian Peter Gay writes in an incisive passage that Kraepelin was one of the "two eminent medical men whom [Freud] regarded as his enemies." The other was Theodor Ziehen in Berlin.[17]

Psychoanalysis caught on quickly in the early twentieth century in America and elsewhere, and an impetus began to develop for the widespread integration of psychoanalysis into clinical treatment. Freud soon became highly esteemed in the West as a man who had uncovered the deep, dark truths about human motivation, desire, disease, and dysfunction. A sharp wedge was driven between organically based psychiatry and Freudian psychiatry as they competed for legitimacy in the modern discourse of mental illness.

The stakes were high. While Kraepelin's Munich clinic struggled financially, so much so that Alzheimer had to foot his own lab costs, Freud and his disciples, including Carl Jung, were achieving widespread adulation for their psychoanalytic system. Their scholarship was also being backed with copious funding.[18] Compared to Kraepelin's expensive organic laboratory, the innovative humanistic techniques of psychoanalysis were ostensibly more effective as well as more cost-efficient.

Kraepelin's push to classify Alzheimer's disease as an organic disorder can be seen in this context as a strategic attempt to gain a foothold in elderly psychosis, a territory that Kraepelin didn't want to lose. His pride, his professional reputation, not to mention his legacy as an academic, were at stake.

Whatever his motivations, when Kraepelin included the label in his *Psychiatry* textbook he set in motion a one-hundred-year history in which the world has gone from one patient tentatively branded with AD to a global epidemic bordering on 25 million.

A TEXTBOOK CASE OF DISEASE CREATION

The philosopher Thomas Kuhn calls medical textbooks the "pedagogic vehicles for the perpetuation of normal science,"[19] which is certainly true in Kraepelin's acceleration of the AD myth.

LIFE AND DEATH AFTER AD

In 1910, with Alzheimer's disease now known among a small number of specialists around the world thanks to Kraepelin, Alzheimer finally became a candidate for a chair in psychiatry. In 1912 he was offered the position of full professor of psychiatry at the Psychiatric Clinic of the Silesian Friedrich Wilhelm University in Breslau. On July 16, Kaiser Wilhelm II personally signed the certificate of appointment, and Alzheimer rose to his chair in psychiatry.

The move fatigued Alzheimer and he became acutely ill on the train journey to Breslau. From the moment he arrived, Alzheimer suffered from exhaustion, experiencing shortness of breath and cardiac palpitations at even the slightest exertion. Lingering symptoms hampered his body, but the doctor, a robust and otherwise vigorous man, still had his mental acuity and pressed on with his work. In addition to directing the clinic and teaching, Alzheimer's duties included work in the pathology institute, consultations, and discussions on cases in pathological anatomy and histology. The many demands of everyday life at the clinic and the pressure to be attentive to administrative details exacted a toll on Alzheimer's health. He suffered increasingly from agonizing chest pains but continued his daily duties. In December 1915, Alzheimer began a rapid decline that vanquished him into a state of bedridden delirium. On Sunday, December 19, 1915, surrounded by his family, Alois Alzheimer died in bed at age fifty-one—the average age of death during that time—of rheumatic heart disease and cardiac failure.

Alzheimer died an accomplished man, with no comprehension of the lasting legacy his discoveries would later earn.

CHAPTER FOUR

THE BIRTH OF THE ALZHEIMER'S EMPIRE

There have been many exciting new discoveries in Alzheimer research at NIH-funded facilities. But this progress cannot continue unless there is a strong and sustained flow of resources for research. I urge Congress to boost federal funds for Alzheimer's research to $1 billion. . . . We could have a serious epidemic on our hands. Alzheimer's is a ticking time bomb in the heads of people in my generation. We must defuse it before it detonates and destroys our minds. Time is running out.

—DAVID HYDE PIERCE, ACTOR AND SPOKESPERSON
FOR THE ALZHEIMER'S ASSOCIATION

For several decades following the publication of Kraepelin's *Psychiatry* text-book, the diagnosis of Alzheimer's disease remained obscure. Its symptoms were mainly attributed to old age, and the medical community did not label patients with "Alzheimer's disease" if it arrived after the sixth decade. The focus shifted from understanding the underlying biology of brain aging to developing bio-psychosocial methods that would better help aging persons and families cope with the challenges posed by cognitive decline.

Though the AD label began to wane, it never vanished completely from medical discourse. As the historian Jesse Ballenger has pointed out, from

1926 to 1935 the *American Journal of Psychiatry* and the *Archives of Neurology and Psychiatry*, the two leading professional journals of American psychiatry and neurology, ran only nine articles concerning Alzheimer's disease.[1] In the middle of the twentieth century, little mention was made of AD, and only a small number of clinicians used the label, reserving it only for patients in their fourth, fifth, or sixth decade who showed the clinical and neuropathological signs of senile dementia.

Pioneers such as the American psychiatrist David Rothschild made it clear that the bleak neuropathologization of aging could be damaging to modern society: "Too exclusive a preoccupation with the cerebral pathology," he argued, had "led to a tendency to forget that the changes are occurring in living, mentally functioning persons."[2] The perils of aging were hard enough without reductionist disease labels like AD making it more difficult to deal with, Rothschild seemed to be saying. He and other psychiatrists of the mid-twentieth century endorsed a bio-psychosocial model of care that normalized brain aging as part of the human condition rather than mythologizing it as a terrorizing disease. They believed not that the pathological substrate of aging was unimportant, but that each individual case required "individual scrutiny, and instead of focusing attention solely on the impersonal tissue process or on more personal influences, the main object should be to estimate the relative importance of these [bio-psychosocial] forces as factors in the origin" of dementia.[3] In many ways, as you will see in Part Three of this book, Rothschild and his colleagues were forerunners to the bio-psychosocial approach to preventing and caring for brain aging that is reemerging at present.

TECHNOLOGY AND THE RESURGENCE OF ALZHEIMER'S

Alzheimer's disease might have remained rare and insignificant if it weren't for several developments in the mid-late twentieth century that gradually increased the mean life expectancy of people living in industrialized countries; namely, the advent of modern medicines, machines, surgical procedures, and, most important, improved diets and sanitation measures that prolonged and protected life. By the late 1960s, thanks to improvements in hygienic and social conditions, and the astounding successes of public-health efforts in controlling epidemics and improving nutrition, an increasing portion of the population began living to eighty-five or older. These so-called old-old persons became the most rapidly growing part of our population. By 1970 the proportion of persons sixty-five and older in the U.S. population had grown to almost 10 percent, up from only 4.3 percent in 1910.[4]

> At present, we not only label those over the age of one hundred as centenarians, but now those over 110 as super-centenarians. . . . What comes next, since the longest lived humans have exceeded 120 years?

As society was becoming populated by men and women who could look forward to longer lives, technical developments in various aspects of neuropathological and biochemical research—for example, electron microscope studies that could zero in on plaques and tangles, neurological imaging devices that could peer into the brain, laboratory procedures that could measure neurotransmitter levels in aging brains—had advanced our ability to study the biology of dementia, paving the way for a return to a more biomedical approach to AD.

The combination of an aging society and the proliferation of technological tools that held the promise of extending old age and relieving its burdens spurred an interest in neurological and gerontological research. Many neuroscientists were among the most avid supporters of the Alzheimer's disease movement and advocated distilling the broad concept of "senile dementia" into discrete categories on the basis of a putative biological cause, as Kraepelin had tried to do a generation before. And, really, who could blame them? The notion that we could relieve the suffering of brain aging appealed to the humanitarian side of many healers. There was also a widely held opinion that a disease called "Alzheimer's" could potentially help remove the stigma of "senility" by targeting a neurobiological condition and taking the onus off the affected senile person. But there was a dark and less benevolent subtext to this movement as well. Some scientists were motivated to bring back Alzheimer's disease as a category because it held the promise of new research grants, potential fame, and the possibility that investment in technology could conquer a major human illness.

THE RISE OF AN EPIDEMIC

In the early 1970s, these neuroscientists, well aware of the aging American culture, began to seek increased funding for their lab work. In order for their research to be taken seriously by those who controlled the public coffers, it was clear that their efforts had to be targeted at something other than the vague process of aging. Their work had to be focused on something real and immediate, something awesome and immanent—a specific disease worthy of massive research efforts into its cause and cure, a "disease of the century." Alzheimer's disease filled that niche perfectly. AD was embraced by the neuroscientific community and formulated in a way that implied that cognitive deterioration and disability in old age were not the result of a natural process, but of a "disease." This marked the revival of the AD myth originated by Kraepelin in 1910.

ALZHEIMER'S BECOMES A NATIONAL INSTITUTION

In 1974 the National Institute on Aging (NIA) was born. Initially, President Richard Nixon vetoed the authorizing bill in an effort to reduce the size of the federal government. Two months before leaving office, he withdrew his opposition, presumably to avoid alienating a Congress that was deliberating his impeachment. The NIA was created and endowed with the responsibility of developing "a plan for a research program on aging designed to coordinate and promote research into the biological, medical, psychological, social, educational, and economic aspects of aging."[5]

Immediately, the NIA, under the leadership of Dr. Robert Butler, a practicing clinical psychiatrist and gerontologist and, to this day, one of my close colleagues, for whom I have enormous respect, began promoting AD as its primary research area, allowing federal funding for the "disease" to be channeled from federal coffers to individual researchers. Butler said, "I decided that we had to make it [Alzheimer's disease] a household word. And the reason I felt that, is that's how the pieces get identified as a national priority. And I call it *the health politics of anguish*."[6]

> ### NIXING THE QUICK FIXING
>
> In the 1970s, Bob Butler confidently predicted that we would fix Alzheimer's in five years. The word *cure* was often used juxtaposed with *AD* in National Institute on Aging statements and fund-raising efforts from other organizations. Needless to say, we've all since been a bit humbled by our inability to understand, treat, or cure the condition. Yet the word *cure* still appears frequently alongside the term *AD*, particularly at fund-raisers.

Butler and the NIA staff were acutely aware of the importance of involving the media in their quest for funding, and, thus, continued efforts were made to keep the press apprised of NIA-sponsored research results and to separate "Alzheimer's disease" from "senility," which Butler considered a "wastebasket term" that rationalized the neglect of the elderly by assuming that cognitive decline was inevitable and irreversible.[7] Zaven Khachaturian, hired by Butler to establish the Neurobiology of Aging program, realized how vital the media would be in spreading and normalizing the disease myth, and put together a systematic strategy for disseminating information to journalists:

> Around here [in Washington] Congress tends to pay more attention to popular media than scientific journals . . . part of the strategy was to inform the public, using the media, about major scientific accomplishments in Alzheimer's disease research and the implications of the scientific findings in terms that lay people could understand.[8]

Advocates for the "disease" surfaced in the media to talk about this new epidemic. The Alzheimer's myth was forming. Dr. Robert Katzman, one of the most notable advocates for AD research, wrote in an April 1976 editorial in a scientific journal that Alzheimer's disease ranked as the fourth or fifth most common cause of death in the United States and called for the country to mobilize resources to address what was a growing social and health problem. Though his claims seemed somewhat exaggerated, Katzman, like other clinicians of his day, effectively questioned the overlaps between normal aging and Alzheimer's disease and challenged the long-held belief of Dr. Alzheimer and others that cognitive decline was an inevitable effect of old age.

Though not everyone was convinced, it became politically incorrect to express personal doubts about whether Alzheimer's disease was a specific form of brain aging. A uniform voice was required to trumpet AD as "abnormal aging" in order to convince politicians and financial backers that this was a disease that could be cured. Nuance was lost, sacrificed on the altar of political expediency. In private, most clinicians and scientists recognized, just as Dr. Alzheimer had done, that some changes in memory and other cognitive functions do occur with aging in all human beings and that the boundaries between normal aging and AD were fuzzy. Still, few were willing to tell the AD emperors that their vestments were a bit more transparent than they thought.

TIME CHANGES, BUT THE LINE IS THE SAME

When I go to Alzheimer's meetings and talk to national and international leaders in the field in private, many express ambivalence about the dominant framework of Alzheimer's disease. Many believe that care deserves greater focus and that the U.S. national Alzheimer's Association is too narrowly focused on biological research. Even state chapter leaders for the Alzheimer's Association express their ambivalence and feel pressured to give "political answers" to the media rather than "honest answers." A colleague of mine once wrote a newspaper column expressing her "political answer" to what the future of Alzheimer's entailed: that the search for the cure is priority number one. However, in a private conversation with a colleague several weeks later, I learned that she had expressed that her "honest answer" was that we need to start investing money in developing new therapeutic interventions for caring for persons with dementia, such as narrative, Reiki, and other complementary and alternative approaches. I found this honesty refreshing, but also disturbing in the sense that this colleague was acknowledging that her professional obligation required her to participate in the distortion and myth making of the AD empire.

It is fair to say that some who fight for the Alzheimer's cause truly believe that it is a specific disease that we can cure. Yet their belief is based on faith in science or clinical intuition more than a reasonable and simple extrapolation of existing knowledge. Many like the colleague mentioned earlier, as well as the one I referred to at the outset of Chapter 2, realize we have created a mythical "monster" that now terrorizes people around the world and distorts our health-care spending. I sometimes tell my friends at the NIH that global warming is a bigger threat than Alzheimer's disease and joke that when the ocean levels rise and flood Washington and the NIH headquarters in Maryland, the "march to progress" against AD will look pretty inconsequential. It's a sardonic joke, of course, but the point about broadening and realigning our priorities is often well taken.

ALZHEIMER'S GOES TO WASHINGTON

In 1979 the Alzheimer's Disease and Related Disorders Association was created in Washington, D.C. After a letter from a family member of an AD victim outlining the problems in caring for someone afflicted with the disease was published in October 1980 in the nationally syndicated newspaper advice column "Dear Abby," the Alzheimer's Disease and Related Disorders Association (ADRDA) received between thirty and forty thousand letters from people in all regions of the United States. The American public, having long accepted cognitive impairment as a component of the aging process, was coming to learn and fear the real scourge of old age, Alzheimer's disease.[9]

In 1982 the ADRDA hired a consulting firm to organize its lobbying efforts to maximize visibility in Washington, increasing its access to representatives and senators. Soon Alzheimer's became a frequent talking point in Congress. On September 15, 1983, the U.S. House of Representatives proposed a resolution declaring November of that year to be National Alzheimer's Disease Month. Congress passed the resolution in the hope that "an increase in the national awareness of the problem of Alzheimer's disease may stimulate the interests and concern of the American people, which may lead, in turn, to increased research and eventually to the discovery of a cure."[10]

The reframing of senility as Alzheimer's disease and the large-scale financial commitments from the government generated excitement among researchers and trickled down to family members and caregivers of Alzheimer's patients, who spoke passionately of its ravages in the mass media and helped shape the contemporary paradigm of AD. Not only did Alzheimer's disease begin to replace senility as a societal marker for cognitive impairments associated with age, a cultural "idiom of distress"[11] also began to emerge around the concept of AD. Alzheimer's acquired dreadful monikers—as the "never-ending funeral," the "mind-robber," the "slow death of the mind," "a loss of selfhood," a "death that leaves the body behind." The disease was consistently personified as a ravaging, marauding, devastating antagonist—a microscopic monster against which science was fighting. Books like the popular *The 36-Hour Day* (Nancy Mace and Peter Rabins, 1981) began to proliferate on bookshelves and became must-reads for patients and caregivers alike. The monstrous myth of Alzheimer's disease was sweeping the country, changing the way we thought about aging. While it was undoubtedly important for the practical challenges of caring for a loved one with progressive cognitive impairment to be recognized by policy makers, the "mythical" aspect of aging—that it is a separate disease that can be cured—has proven ultimately to be destructive.

By 1985 the NIA had established ten Alzheimer's Disease Research Centers (ADRCs) across the country. I was affiliated with the NIA's ADRC at Johns Hopkins University, where I developed clinic programs and a Brain Resource Center. The government passed a law authorizing the NIA director to make grants specifically for AD-related research—the first such disease-specific mandate in public-health law. By 1984, Alzheimer's Disease International (ADI), a confederation of all the national Alzheimer's groups, was founded with encouragement from the World Health Organization.

I have attended most of ADI's meetings around the world for the last twenty years, and at the 2006 meeting in Berlin I spoke and moderated a debate on whether Alzheimer's disease is an outmoded concept. This international group provides an important global perspective on the impact of dementia. The increasing challenges of aging populations in developing countries deserve greater emphasis on the world stage.

A "CAUSE CELEBRITY"

The mainstream acceptance of the AD myth and the emergence of a cultural language of distress and fear about AD was further augmented by celebrity involvement with the emerging "cause." Princess Yasmin Aga Khan, the daughter of film star Rita Hayworth—who had been diagnosed with AD in 1981—was a highly visible advocate for the disease. When her mother, the world-famous "Love Goddess," died on May 14, 1987, Yasmin Khan released the doctors from their confidentiality obligations, ensuring that her famous mother would make the term *Alzheimer's disease* known throughout the world. This surging public awareness was only reinforced by the stunning revelation in 1994 that Ronald Reagan had developed AD.

FAMOUS PEOPLE AFFECTED BY ALZHEIMER'S

Charles Bronson—actor

Winston Churchill—prime minister of Great Britain

Perry Como—singer

Aaron Copland—composer

Willem de Kooning—artist

Ralph Waldo Emerson—writer

Barry Goldwater—U.S. senator from Arizona

William Hanna—animator (Hanna-Barbera)

Charlton Heston—actor

Juliana Wilhelmina—queen of the Netherlands

Beatrice Lillie—comedian

Jack Lord—actor

Burgess Meredith—actor

Iris Murdoch—novelist and philosopher

Otto Preminger—director

Maurice Ravel—composer

Ronald Reagan—U.S. president

Sugar Ray Robinson—boxer

Norman Rockwell—artist

Margaret Rutherford—actress

Robert Sargent Shriver—politician

Cyrus Vance—secretary of state

E. B. White—writer

Reagan's continued advocacy of AD research throughout the 1980s and 1990s helped aim an even more acute spotlight on Alzheimer's disease and led to the 1990s being declared "The Decade of the Brain" by his vice president, George H. W. Bush. In 1979 the NIA had spent approximately $4 million on research into AD; by 1991 it was spending $155 million—a thirty-seven-fold increase.[12] In 2007 federal research funding for the "War on AD" swelled to an astonishing $643 million. One can only imagine how Alois Alzheimer—who himself concluded that there was "no tenable reason to consider [his] cases as caused by a specific disease process"—would have reacted had he been alive to see the enormous financial backing against a disease bearing his name in the latter decades of the twentieth century.

THE METAMORPHOSIS OF A DISEASE LABEL

In my career, the terminology for cognitive impairments associated with brain aging has evolved from "senility" to "senile dementia" to "senile dementia of the Alzheimer's type" to "Alzheimer's disease and related disorders" to "Alzheimer's disease." What's next? It's up to us to decide.

DIGGING DEEPER INTO THE DOMINANT METAPHORS OF ALZHEIMER'S DISEASE

The myth of Alzheimer's disease is now deeply embedded in our culture, and thus the dominant metaphors that serve as its pillars appear in our everyday language. Thanks to the framework shaped by the AD empire— the constituent Alzheimer's advocacy organizations, the pharmaceutical industry, and self-interested researchers—over the last three decades, our generation has come to think of late-stage brain aging as "a disease called

Alzheimer's" that "robs" and "ravages" the minds of elderly individuals like a foreign invader and must be defeated by science in a long protracted struggle—a "War on Alzheimer's." And indeed, when we talk about Alzheimer's, our language, like a social reflex, invariably drifts back to military metaphors (italics below added for emphasis).

In 2004, Paul and Terry Klassen, founders of Sunrise Senior Living, wrote, "Recognizing and addressing the needs of America's families with Alzheimer's is *a critical battle in our overall war on Alzheimer's.*"[13] The mission statement of the Alzheimer's Association states, in part, that they have: "The compassion to care, the *leadership to conquer.*"[14] Peruse their Web site closer and you'll read that "Alzheimer's disease is a progressive brain disorder that *gradually destroys a person's memory* and ability to learn, reason, make judgments, communicate and carry out daily activities."[15] In the 2005 *Newsweek* special issue on health, the magazine reported that researchers are "*mounting direct assaults* on the underlying disease process" and later explained that "Alzheimer's is a *progressive, devastating, and incurable* illness."[16] Similarly, in an article entitled "Small, but Promising, Advance in War Against Alzheimer's: From Drugs to Vaccines, Progress Is Reported," the November 21, 2003, *Health Day Reporter* wrote: "Alzheimer's is a *horribly intractable* disease. But *the fight against the mind-wasting ailment has been marked by a recent series of encouraging, albeit incremental, advances.*" It's not just the media. It's also the medical profession. In the foreword to a caregiver's book about the disease, a physician writes, "*This illness strikes at the very core of our being . . . rob[bing] the victims of their unique thought processes, their insights, their judgment, their ability to learn new information.*"[17]

The very notion of being diagnosed with AD strikes abject terror in all of us who have all-too-susceptible aging minds. It also changes our relationship to those who are labeled with the disease. Instead of simply being persons with aging brains they become "Alzheimer's victims," diseased, demented, and stigmatized.

Further, by invoking a war, the media and the AD empire imply potential victory, causing us to readily assume that the cognitive loss that characterizes old age (and has done so for all human beings throughout man's 2.6-million-year history) will be *fixed* by human intervention. As we have seen, researchers, the drug industry, and AD activist organizations benefit greatly from this particular framing, telling the public that a victory will be won by science and waging a "fight for the cure" that implies progressive victory. People like Zaven Khachaturian, my colleague formerly of the NIA and now an independent consultant, continue to mesmerize us with quotes like this: "Those of us in the front lines of the fight against Alzheimer's have never been closer to unmasking this mysterious thief, the robber of the very thing that makes human beings unique."[18]

THE ART OF MINDFUL RESISTANCE

The Buddha taught that "we are what we think. All that we are arises with our thoughts. With our thoughts, we make the world." And indeed, the dominant metaphors of the Alzheimer's framework pervade the thought processes of millions upon millions of human beings, profoundly influencing their self-image as they age. Those of us unlucky enough to be given an AD diagnosis are transformed into diseased individuals, while the rest of us simply wait in fear of acquiring the disease, or dread the possibility of loved ones being labeled, with the hope that science can somehow win the battle.

Following the Buddha's wisdom, we must change our thought process about brain aging. Reflect on the words and images that come to mind when you think of Alzheimer's disease. And then think about them in the larger context of the knowledge you now have about the biology and history of AD. Questioning the foundations of your current thoughts about AD can help you shape a new framework for brain aging.

While millions of "AD victims" are created by the label each year, substantial amounts of public and private resources are devoted to winning the war on the disease. Consequently, our war chest is expended on the fight for a cure instead of on diplomacy—preventive medicine that could be aimed at keeping brains cognitively fit for a lifetime, and caregiving infrastructure that could help families and communities better adapt to the inevitable changes that accompany brain aging.

WHO BENEFITS FROM THIS AGGRESSIVE MEDICALIZATION OF BRAIN AGING?

Many of those in the Alzheimer's empire appreciate that the world of dementia is more complicated than they often state publicly—they know, and even express in their private conversations with one another and with me, that there is no singular disease called "AD," and that it is a complex, scientifically imprecise social construct that may never be cured.

My colleagues in the AD empire are using language that is beginning to diverge from the standard line. In a radio interview on NPR (November 16, 2006), John Hardy, a molecular biologist from the NIH and an old friend of mine, was paired up with me to debate whether we were putting too much money into finding a cure. In large part, we both agreed that there was excessive hype about a cure and that the dominance of profit making led to these unrealistic claims for quick fixes. Later in the debate, the interviewer asked us whether we would ever have an "absolute" cure. To my mind, a cure is by definition absolute; it implies that the condition is eradicated so that no trace is left, which I find to be an implausible scenario for AD. Interestingly, John agreed that an absolute cure was unlikely in part because of the association between Alzheimer's and aging. Will the less responsible members of the Alzheimer empire (of which John is not one) now back off and claim that we are only fighting to find a "relative" cure, and that there are other priorities—namely, care and prevention—that deserve our attention and investment?

By perpetuating the notion of a war on AD, invoking imagery of a battlefield of infirmity and disorder, and imagining their organizations as being on the front lines in the fight against AD, organizations such as the Alzheimer's Association and the National Institute on Aging receive hundreds of millions of dollars of support from citizens and taxpayers. While this is not a conspiracy, it's a clever business and politically motivated strategy executed by organizations that know how to tell compelling stories with vivid language that will help sustain themselves.

War imagery has a special power over the human psyche; it instills a sense of fear and urgency that prompts rapid action. It also provides cartes blanches for whoever declares the war. In light of the AD empire's fund-raising strategy, which takes the form of an ongoing war, we might well draw wisdom from George Orwell's cautionary words that "war is not meant to be won. It is meant to be continuous." Indeed, an escalating war necessitates escalating funds. And escalating funds mean expanded resources and ongoing survival for organizations.

> I have great respect for current Alzheimer's leadership at the NIA. I suspect we will see a shift in their position on brain aging in years to come, and a greater focus on nonbiological approaches.

Speaking of business plans, the pharmaceutical industry is more than happy to play off the health anxieties of the population and supply the fire-power in the medical arms race against AD. After all, you and every other aging person who fears Alzheimer's or is given the diagnosis are potential drug consumers. Researchers such as myself are given generous grants to study the enemy and to use sophisticated technology to test its weaknesses and to develop potential silver bullets. Many of us are flown around the world by drug companies who pamper us, wine and dine us, and try to co-opt us into endorsing their products so that their markets can expand. As of Spring 2007, I have carried out my last consulting obligations and will accept no more consulting money directly from drug companies.

As I mentioned, the mass media also plays a fundamental role in disseminating the war metaphors. By quoting experts who offer words of encouragement using complex (and often bellicose) medical terminology, and by enthusiastically publicizing new neuroimaging devices and pharmaceuticals, the mass media legitimizes, informs, and helps shape the myth of

Alzheimer's disease that we have all come to know. I've seen this phenomenon progressively unfold over my last three decades in the field and deeply regret the effect it has had on the public.

THE LIMITS OF OUR INVESTMENTS

Interestingly, my wealthier patients provide some of the most profound lessons about the limits of money in winning the battle against AD. They tend to read the newspapers and are aware of the latest stories about therapeutic efforts, and are thus willing and ready to try the latest front-line treatments.

One of my most interesting situations involved a billionaire who gave me a multithousand-dollar grant to search the world for a memory enhancer, hoping that a powerful pill might just be waiting to be found in some foreign pharmacopeia somewhere. Though I searched high and low, and consulted with dozens of trusted friends on many continents, I was not so surprisingly unable to locate any miracle pills. His case merely reinforces the point that with so-called Alzheimer's disease, money cannot buy a cure.

THE "WAR ON PERSONHOOD"

Besides the military metaphors of AD, equally disturbing is language that would have us believe Alzheimer's disease causes us to "lose ourselves" to the disease. One need look no further than the titles of some of the most popular Alzheimer's books and articles to see the pervasive reach of this metaphor: *The Loss of Self* by Donna Cohen and Carl Eisdorfer; *Losing My Mind: An Intimate Look at Life with Alzheimer's* by Thomas DeBaggio; *Death in Slow Motion: A Memoir of a Daughter, Her Mother, and the Beast Called Alzheimer's* by Eleanor Cooney.

The usage of these metaphors by the authors is quite understandable. Dementia *does* alter identity. When we watch our loved ones cognitively age we fear that there will be a living, breathing body present, but that the person we have known and loved will turn into a non-person without personality at all. The framing of this metaphor goes as follows: Once a person loses the ability to connect to the past and future in a meaningful way, they lose themselves.

But just like the military metaphor, the loss-of-self metaphors so prevalent in our cultural discourse give us the harmful impression that just because the individual's awareness of their own identity has been seriously "damaged," identity itself is "destroyed." A person's identity is thus equated with the raw "meat" of their brain such that when that organ is injured or even reduced in size, so is their humanity. A mind-set of fatalism sets in, causing us to write our loved ones off and lament their progressive decline as we understand their condition through the loss-of-self metaphor.

As I expressed earlier, cognition and rationality must not be equated with personhood. This viewpoint, which the late Tom Kitwood called the "malignant social psychology" of dementia, often precludes the empathetic engagement that persons who are aging deserve. Perhaps their cognitive decline is an invitation to us to return to more primordial aspects of our being that attune us to the rhythms of the body and its functions. Perhaps by venturing to engage with our aging loved ones instead of treating them as diseased we can even learn a great deal about ourselves, and what it means to be a person.[19] Perhaps we can use it as an opportunity to improve our nonverbal communication skills, our caregiving skills, and enjoy our immediate sensory experiences in a more relaxed fashion. Perhaps it can even call up a wellspring of energy and compassion that is more healing than any pharmaceutical pill. As Kitwood wrote a decade ago: "Dementia will always have a deeply tragic aspect, both for those who are affected and for those who are close to them. There is, however, a vast difference between a tragedy, in which persons are actively involved and morally committed, and a blind and hopeless submission to fate."[20] The story we tell can either amplify the magnitude of the "tragedy," or soften and normalize it while putting the prevailing emphasis on interdependence and compassion.

MOVING FORWARD WITH THE WISDOM OF T. S. ELIOT

People with cognitive dysfunction will suffer enough as it is without us reducing them to being "disease victims." Instead of leading the fight in an unwinnable war, and leaving legions of fallen AD victims who have "lost their selves," the AD empire must now help people think and speak differently about brain aging in a way that nurtures an ethical commitment to our emerging elders.

> ### CHANGING THE MYTH OF ALZHEIMER'S HERE AND ABROAD
>
> Part of my efforts to end Alzheimer's has involved me talking to leaders of AD organizations around the world and encouraging them to adapt their organizational names to be less disease-oriented. My friends Harry Cayton (the former head of the Alzheimer's Society in the U.K. and current patient advocate in the National Health Service), Henry Brodaty (who is the former chairman of Alzheimer's Disease International), and Steve Rudin (former head of the Alzheimer's Society in Canada) have been actively involved in attempting to reimagine their organizations in light of the new reality we face. In Canada the Alzheimer's Society hands out shirts that read "The Story Is Changing." And across the world it certainly is. However, the attempt to improve upon the framework of the AD myth is not easy. As Upton Sinclair famously wrote, "It is difficult to get a man to understand something when his salary depends on his not understanding it."

Increasingly, colleagues in the field have been telling me that my message resonates with them. The grounds are fertile for a new story of brain aging, and the AD empire can be a powerful force in shaping a new paradigm of cognitive decline in the twenty-first century. They can be allies rather than adversaries.

There's a famous story about T. S. Eliot delivering a philosophical lecture on a serious moral problem at a renowned American university. After making his speech, Eliot opened up the floor to questions from the audience. Immediately, an undergraduate began waving his hand back and forth to draw the poet's attention. When called upon, the student stood and asked, "Mr. Eliot, what are we going to do about this problem you have discussed?"

"My dear sir," Eliot responded, "you have asked the wrong question. You must understand that in life we face two kinds of problems. One kind demands your question, 'What are we going to do about it?' The other calls for a different question, 'How does one behave towards it?' "[21]

Eliot's point was that human beings often seem to have an innate drive to conquer and subdue the problems in the world for which we lack answers. The type of question asked by the student, which demands a purely technical, instrumental response aimed at conquering a problem, is the type of question the AD empire poses about brain aging: How are we going to fix Alzheimer's? How will we defeat the "monster"? In contrast, the second type of question put forth by Eliot is far more subtle. It allows a wider range of postures to the "problem" at hand, including judging the situation not a problem at all. This approach seeks peaceful coexistence with that which is unknown and poses a deeper range of challenges that no particular policies, strategies, devices, or weapons are expected to eradicate. How we frame phenomena in our world, Eliot suggested, is vital to how we construe our reality.

I do not deny that suffering occurs with what we now call Alzheimer's. But as psychiatrists such as David Rothschild noted over a half-century ago, if suffering cannot be eliminated, it can be ameliorated. Human words and concepts embedded in our personal relationships can enhance suffering or reduce it. I only claim that how we use the AD label can often compound human suffering and distort our priorities, and that changing the way we think about and speak about brain aging can enrich our experience of it.

> I have no intention of having committed people in Alzheimer's organizations lose their jobs. My point is, rather, that we need to prioritize the right jobs and get to work, for the task of rising up to meet the challenges of our aging world is enormous.

Instead of declaring a war against brain aging and the loss of selfhood, and promising a quick fix for Alzheimer's disease, we must move beyond these facile and misleading assertions and begin asking how we are going to behave toward it. It is unlikely that we will ever be able to "fix" what we now call Alzheimer's disease. Quite simply, it is not a real war. The struggle will rage on interminably, with casualties suffered by those unfortunate enough to be labeled with an incurable "disease" and their families. Since much of the commentary and information that makes its way into our media coverage and into our pharmaceutical educational materials is provided by organizations in the AD empire, the leaders of these influential institutions have the power and the means necessary to guide the public in thinking differently about their aging and shift the paradigm of the "disease." As many of us leaders in the AD field grow older, our need to "cure" Alzheimer's may be softened into a need to accept and embrace the mystery and the awe of the brain-aging process and to help others do the same. As my departed colleague Tom Kitwood so eloquently put it: There is a place for continued genetic research but not genetic hype; there is a place for neuropathology, but not neuropathic ideology.[22]

Just before Tom passed away, he visited Cleveland. Over lunch at a local hospice, he shared with me the story of an atheist physician with dementia whose last words to Tom were, "I think I have seen the soul." Profound revelations about ourselves and others can emerge from the suffering associated with dementia.

A new story that is more sensitive to suffering individuals and honest about the limits of science can promote the quality of life for all of us who are aging in the twenty-first century. Indeed, imagining new stories that include a recognition of the limits of science and our human capabilities will allow us richer and deeper appreciation of how our brain works, what aging means, and how we need to celebrate our common humanity and recognize our responsibilities to future generations.

PART TWO

SCIENCE AND TREATMENT

CHAPTER FIVE

Waiting for Godot: Alzheimer's Treatments Past and Present

When a lot of remedies are suggested for a disease, that means it can't be cured.

—Anton Chekhov

Americans now spend more than $200 billion a year on prescription drugs, and the largest consumers are senior citizens. Our faith in the pharmaceutical industry is powerful. We rarely pause to think: What exactly are loved ones with memory challenges putting into their bodies? How were our current drugs developed? How much can we expect of them, and of the stem cell treatments and amyloid vaccines we hear bruited about with such promise? Are there complementary and alternative treatments that offer more promise? We must think deeply and thoughtfully about these questions to put drug development in proper historical and social context.

For years, people recommended that I read Samuel Beckett's play *Waiting for Godot*. So a couple years ago I picked a copy up and had a read. It's a surreal tale that follows two vagabonds who wait interminably in a field for the arrival of someone named Godot, who they hope will save them. As the days while away, these two men take turns convincing each other that Godot will soon arrive, although despite their hopeful outlooks, they are inwardly panicked that the man will never show. The profound tragedy of the play is that as Godot fails to appear, we realize that the two wayward men are victims of false hope. They have invested their time and resources in service of an illusion.

I see a meaningful link between Beckett's play and our current predicament with Alzheimer's disease. When the lay organizations, biotech firms, pharmaceutical marketing departments, media, and other profiteering players in the AD empire implore us to give them just a little more money and a little more time to produce a miracle cure for AD, we are waiting for Godot—investing our resources, our time, and our hope in the pursuit of a cure that may never arrive for a disease that we cannot diagnose or effectively treat.

> *Look, if we doubled our research output it would halve the amount of time it will take to find a cure.*
> —THE LATE DR. LEON THAL, FORMER DIRECTOR OF
> THE ALZHEIMER'S DISEASE RESEARCH CENTER
> AT THE UNIVERSITY OF CALIFORNIA, SAN DIEGO

Hope is perhaps the most important commodity in the world, for it allows us to get up every morning and face the challenges of each day. It creates an expectation that the future will be better for us and our children. But is there really hope for curing Alzheimer's disease in the near future? Or is it hype?

We must remember that multimillion-dollar organizations like the Alzheimer's Association and other private foundations, as well as the Alzheimer's programs at the National Institute on Aging and in universities, which collectively house hundreds and hundreds of employees, would not be able to sustain their funding if Alzheimer's disease did not exist as a cause. Nor would drug companies find the path to profits so clearly marked if cognitive dysfunction were considered a natural outgrowth of the aging process rather than a pathological condition called Alzheimer's disease or Mild Cognitive Impairment that could be treated with pills.

THE NUMBERS DON'T "AD" UP

In 2004 a conference organized by the International Psychogeriatrics Association was held in Washington to gather consensus on the clinical usage of MCI. During the conference, Henry Brodaty, a friend and colleague of mine, and I tried to point out the social and cultural difficulties with the use of the label. After the conference ended, we polled participants (all experts who were invested in the concept of MCI) as to whether the term *MCI* should currently be used clinically. Only 57 percent of those polled answered yes. The results probably should not have been so surprising. People in the AD field may be a bit more honest when guaranteed anonymity.

For such organizations as these, Alzheimer's is their raison d'être, the foundation from which they draw financial nourishment and sustenance. Hyperbole is extremely useful for maintaining funding.[1] As long as our culture is convinced that there is a cure waiting to be found for a condition classified as Alzheimer's disease, these organizations will never cease to exist. This is why it is so important that they drill the conventional myth of AD into our minds and promise us that "new treatments are on the horizon."[2]

The American Alzheimer's Association has understandably led the world looking for a cure. After all, it is in the United States where much of the research is conducted. This association has had a dual mission of finding the cure and improving care, but increasingly it has lost the balance between these approaches, and is out of step with other national organizations around the world that recognize the limits of science and the need to improve care and prevention in the present.

SPREAD THE WEALTH FOR HEALTH

Both the Alzheimer's Association and National Institute on Aging attend to the psychosocial aspects of dementia but only to a minor degree relative to the quest for biological fixes. Through the years I have tried to encourage the growth of research into nonpharmacological approaches to brain aging such as psychosocial and educational interventions and even other so-called complementary and alternative therapies. Although these efforts have paid off with more attention being focused on nonpharmacological methods, there is still a sense of tokenism to these organizations' efforts to support care rather than cure. The fact that the lion's share of the research budget is being allocated to Alzheimer's research has caused some of my colleagues, especially gerontologists, to complain about the dominance of Alzheimer's disease in the NIA budget. For example, Richard Miller, a prominent researcher at the University of Michigan, wrote an editorial complaining about the "Alzheimerization" of the NIA. In personal conversations, even Robert Butler laments the exaggerated emphasis.

Although we'd all like to see more effective treatments for the ravages of brain aging, the current framing of AD exists to too great a degree for the political and economic gain of individuals and organizations, rather than the benefit of individual patients, their families, and society's needs at large. It stretches the truth and builds false hope for many millions of people who are undergoing real suffering. As we labor under the misapprehension that a single condition called "Alzheimer's disease" exists, and wait patiently for a cure, funds flow freely into the pockets of those who distort the truth. It's manipulative, unfair, and unwise. AD supporters are entitled to their opinion about the promise of science, but we must allow other voices, which are growing in amplitude, to express alternative interpretations of the current science. How much longer do we endure and invest in the wait for a "breakthrough"? How much can we improve upon current treatments? And in anticipating a cure for Alzheimer's, are we, too, waiting for Godot?

CHOLINESTERASE INHIBITORS: JUST HOW GOOD ARE THEY?

Currently, the FDA has approved four pills called cholinesterase inhibitors for persons with mild to moderate dementia, and recently one for severe dementia as well. Cholinesterase is an enzyme found primarily at nerve endings that catalyzes the hydrolysis, or decomposition, of acetylcholine. Acetylcholine is a neurotransmitter, one of the chemicals that shuttle between nerve cells in the brain, and is essential for learning and memory.

As our research at Johns Hopkins in the 1980s revealed, the loss of cholinergic (meaning "producing-acetylcholine") nerve cells in a part of the brain called the cholinergic basal forebrain (also known as the sub-stantia innominata or nucleus basalis of Meynert) is associated with the symptoms of dementia. As I mentioned earlier, the cholinergic forebrain sends its axons, or connections, widely through other parts of the brain including the cortex, the most advanced part of the brain where most of our complex thinking goes on, and the hippocampus, which, as you know, is critical for creating new memories. Cell death in the basal fore-brain can lead to widespread depletion of acetylcholine throughout the brain and is one of the correlates of the loss in memory and learning ca-pability.

We still don't know exactly why these cholinergic nerve cells in the basal forebrain die, or how to prevent their death. So instead of addressing that problem, current treatments focus on inhibiting cholinesterase, the en-zyme that breaks down acetylcholine in the brain. Because we are unable to stop the death of acetylcholine-producing cells, the rationale goes, we should preserve levels of the already-existing neurotransmitter. The family of FDA-approved cholinesterase inhibitors (ChEIs)—tacrine (Cognex), donepezil (Aricept), rivastigmine (Exelon), and galantamine (Razadyne)—was created as a result of this research, which came to be known as "the cholinergic hypothesis."

GETTING A READ ON THE DRUGS
AVAILABLE TODAY

Tacrine is the only one of the four cholinesterase inhibitors not used much today because it has to be administered four times a day and was shown to cause liver inflammation in many people.

For the other currently available cholinesterase inhibitors, there are two primary questions of relevance:

1. Do they improve quality of life?
2. Are they cost-effective?

The answer to the first question is a very guarded yes for some people, and a clear no for others. Although cholinesterase inhibitors demonstrate small improvements on cognitive and global function in some patients with mild to moderate AD, and may work in some severe cases as well, they do not work for others, and can have side effects that include gastrointestinal upset, nausea, vomiting, diarrhea, and muscle cramps as well as sleep disturbances, insomnia, and nightmares.

MY EXPERIENCE ON (AD) DRUGS

In 2002 I decided to take donepezil myself. Since the potential for cognitive enhancement intrigued me, and because many of my patients were on donepezil, I began my own pill regimen under careful supervision, and attempted to assess its effects. After a few days I began to feel nauseated and this queasiness led me to stop taking the drug before we could fully assess the effects. I also had some quite entertaining but also disconcerting dreams that likely were by-products of the drug. It made me wonder if many of the elderly individuals whom I had prescribed cholinesterase inhibitors for feel the same side effects I did, but, because of their dementia, lack the ability to articulate their discomfort. At any rate, the experience reinforced my ambivalence about giving my patients these drug treatments.

The side effects result from the pervasiveness of acetylcholine in other parts of our bodies, especially in our hearts and gastrointestinal systems. If you inhibit cholinesterase to the benefit of the brain, it may detrimentally affect other systems, perhaps speeding up the gastrointestinal system or the heart. In fact, two recent studies of cholinesterase inhibitors in people with vascular disease raised concern about high mortality rates in those taking ChEI drugs, and also raised the issue of long-term safety of patients who may be at higher risk for heart problems or other serious side effects.[3] Although this risk population is small, and most people suffer relatively few side effects as a result of taking the medications, the positive effects are often very subtle and barely noticeable. I have struggled over the years with prescribing pills that I worry confer relatively little benefit, come at a high cost, subject a patient to possible side effects, and for which we have insufficient data on long-term safety. Still, I believe it is important for me to give families the choice of opting for the pills.

SAFETY FIRST: "DO NO HARM"

In many cases, although drugs are FDA-approved we do not have adequate long-term safety data. Deaths have been reported in studies of vascular dementia with donepezil, galantamine, and other drugs, particularly neuroleptics (antipsychotics), for behavioral symptoms in elderly patients taking them. It is often difficult to know if an apparent increase in deaths in a drug study represents a deviation from chance. After all, many older people are enrolled in such studies and a certain percentage will die unrelated to any drug effect. Nevertheless, we desperately need a better post-FDA approval surveillance system to track the long-term dangers of drugs. We also need to focus on developing more behavioral therapies for the aggression and depression we sometimes see in persons with late-stage brain aging. Instead of pumping individuals with neuroleptics and antidepressants, we must begin integrating new humanistic therapies into our mainstream armature of care: narrative therapies, music therapies, art therapies, pet therapies, and other forms of therapies that engage people with other human beings and with nature. Too often, we fail to see the enormous healing potential in basic human connection, although that has been the single most effective intervention our ancestors have used to care for one another for generations upon generations.

In practice it is difficult to know if reported initial improvement in some individuals is due to the drug or the placebo effect. After someone has been on a drug for a while it is difficult to get them off it, because even though the medication is having little effect, patients do not want to run the risk of getting worse. In my own practice, I advise the patient and family about possible risks and benefits of ChEIs, but have decided recently to try to leave the actual prescription to the primary-care doctor.

OVERMEDICATION NATION

One major problem in our health-care system today is polypharmacy. This is the name geriatricians use to describe a situation in which a person is taking multiple drugs that interact with each other to produce negative effects. There is even a condition called "iatrogenic drug-related confusional state," which results from the long-term buildup of drugs in a person's body. *If you do choose to go on ChEI treatments, you must make sure your physician is aware of other medications you are taking.* Drugs such as antipsychotics, anti-epileptics, tranquilizers, muscle relaxants (such as alprazolam, clonazepam, diazepam, and triazolam), and overactive-bladder drugs (such as oxybutynin, tolterodine, and trospium) may induce dementia-like symptoms over the long term.

It is better if one doctor coordinates all the medicines. Primary-care doctors tend not to be impressed by the therapeutic effects of the currently available antidementia drugs, a feeling I share. Drug companies expend enormous amounts of effort and cash to get opinion leaders like myself to convince doctors in the trenches to use their medications. At stake is the credibility of specialists, who must stand up for their patients and not answer to the powerful empire of the drug industry.

DRUGS COST TOO DARN MUCH

Why do drugs cost four dollars a day for the individual consumer? Why doesn't our government get to negotiate lower prices through Medicare as is done through the Veterans Administration, for example? The simple answer is that landmark legislation—the Medicare Bill Part D—was passed by Congress in 2003 to prevent this and to ensure that millions of taxpayer dollars would be spent on drugs. The fact that this bill was passed in the early-morning hours (perhaps so C-SPAN viewers would not be watching), surrounded by hundreds of pharmaceutical lobbyists (who, according to some observers, wrote much of the bill), and that many of the major politicians and staffers who pushed the bill through the legislative process ended up working for the industry is a national disgrace. But laws can be changed and we must encourage our politicians to stand up to the powerful drug industry just as we exhort our doctors to do the same.

Given that the pharmaceutical industry is supposedly a prime example of the success of global capitalism, driven by a competitive market for drugs, why do we not see more price competition? Some aggressive competition occurs in the closed-door negotiations between industry and such large purchasers of drugs as health maintenance and other organizations. For my individual patients who pay out of pocket, there appears to be relatively little variation in price among the drugs. I would like to see lower prices through a combination of genuine competition and more balanced information about the effects, for good and ill, of drugs available to consumers and the market.

Each of the FDA-approved drugs costs approximately four dollars a day if the patient pays out of pocket, which adds up to nearly $1,500 a year. This is an enormous cost for individuals, especially when the effects of ChEIs are so marginal in most cases. I sympathize with the need of my patients to find a biological pill treatment for their condition, but as a clinician committed to minimizing human suffering and promoting quality of life, I will not enthusiastically prescribe medicines I no longer believe provide value for the money. Nor do I feel it is worth spending so much time talking about drugs with patients and families in the clinic when there are more important topics to be considered in the precious little time we have together.

THE NEW DRUG ON THE BLOCK

A more recent addition to the list of FDA-approved drugs, memantine (Namenda), created some initial excitement and hope, in part because it acts through a different mechanism than cholinesterase inhibitors. Memantine's action involves the inhibition of glutamate, one of the most ubiquitous neurotransmitters in the cerebral cortex and in the nervous system in general.

An excitatory amino acid neurotransmitter, glutamate's usual function is to stimulate neurons to fire more frequently. At Johns Hopkins, I studied the role of glutamate in cognition and made some effort to measure its receptors in the human brain. With acetylcholine, too little of the neurotransmitter has clear detrimental consequences on attention and memory and higher levels can improve cognition, but the situation with glutamate is murkier. Experimental research in animals has shown that if glutamate receptors are overstimulated by the abundance of glutamate, neurons may die. Recall from Chapter 2 that this research is based on the excitatory hypothesis.

A new story has emerged that argues the nerve cell death occurring in a variety of degenerative diseases, including Alzheimer's disease and Huntington's disease, occurs because nerve cells are stimulated to death—shorted out—by an overabundance of glutamate-producing action. Memantine acts as a glutamate receptor antagonist that blocks the effects of glutamate. Thus, the companies that make memantine brand their product to make doctors believe that their drug slows the biological progression of the illness by preventing cell death. However, beneath the marketing pitch, there is no clinical evidence to demonstrate this effect.

There are side effects to memantine that are usually manageable, but can include headache, constipation, dizziness, and agitation. Despite its promise, memantine does not appear to constitute a significant upgrade over the other ChEIs. I would not dissuade patients from trying it but would put a definite check on the expectations they might have for a miraculous turn-around.

Interestingly, in 2006 the National Institute for Health and Clinical Excellence (NICE) in the United Kingdom recommended that memantine not be reimbursed by the British government for any patients with Alzheimer's. In fact, cholinesterase inhibitors were only approved for persons diagnosed as having moderate disease. While a controversial decision, it did represent a systematic attempt by the British government to decide which medications are really worth paying for by taxpayers. The reasons why memantine was not approved in Britain are complex, but apparently relate in part to the inconsistency in trial results and the drug's limited effect.

IS THERE HOPE FOR FUTURE CHOLINERGIC DRUGS?

The story of cholinergic drugs is by no means over. Although the benefits of current drugs are not what we had hoped for, there may be other ways to improve our ability to pharmacologically enhance the functioning of the cholinergic basal forebrain system, which, you might remember from Chapter 2, sends its axons throughout the brain, distributing acetylcholine to various brain regions, including the hippocampus.

MY HISTORY WITH NICOTINIC RECEPTORS

As a researcher at Johns Hopkins in the 1980s, when my colleagues and I described the loss of cells in the cholinergic basal forebrain, I started working as a research fellow in our basic neuroscience department to learn about neurotransmitter receptors and how to measure them. Acetylcholine binds to two broad classes of cholinergic receptors—muscarinic and nicotinic—named for drugs that bind particularly strongly to these two major types. Most other investigators had been examining the muscarinic receptors because they were more common in the central nervous systems and easier to measure. We were the first to point out that the nicotinic receptors were the most affected in AD and related cholinergic dementias, while muscarinic receptors do not seem to change much. This prompted us to look at drugs that might stimulate nicotinic receptors.

Surprisingly, a promising future avenue of research involves one of the most deadly products ever used by human beings: tobacco. One of the active ingredients in tobacco is nicotine, which, as any smoker will tell you, delivers an immediate cognitive boost. This sharpening of arousal and attention may be due to the fact that we have various subtypes of nicotinic cholinergic receptors in the neuronal synapses in our brains that are stimulated by compounds such as nicotine and acetylcholine. When stimulated, the nicotinic receptors allow the passage of ions into the neuron that initiates cell firing in certain cell populations that keep us more alert. Nicotinic responses tend to be fast-onset, short in duration, and excitatory in their nature, but nicotine itself is addictive. Nevertheless, this boosting action offers a biological basis for developing drugs that would act selectively on certain types of nicotinic receptor sites, potentially providing the benefits of cognitive enhancement without the safety and addiction concerns associated with the nicotine in tobacco.

Understanding how drugs might work requires a closer look at the nicotinic receptor site. Located in the synapses of our neurons, nicotinic receptors are composed of five "gateway" polypeptide subunits arranged circularly in an ion-gated channel. Once stimulated, they allow ion particles to travel through the gateway from the outside to the inside of the cell, in turn causing the cell to "fire" its message and activate other cells. Two kinds of subtypes of nicotinic receptors are called alpha 4/beta 2 and alpha 7, based on the proteins that make up the five-unit circle. These may be particularly important subtypes to stimulate with drugs because of their association with cognitive activity. Tellingly, these subtypes of nicotinic receptors are found in the hippocampus, a structure we know is important for memory. One of my final consulting engagements with the pharmaceutical industry was with a company called Targacept (a spin-off company from the R. J. Reynolds Tobacco Co.), which is currently developing drugs to target these subtypes of nicotinic receptors. Right now they have several candidate drugs that might succeed in the goal of providing some greater symptomatic benefit to patients with Alzheimer's disease and related conditions through action on nicotinic cholinergic receptors.

Over the years, I have worked with academic colleagues, and with a va-

NICOTINIC RECEPTORS HERE, THERE, AND EVERYWHERE

Nicotinic receptors are not only found in the brain, they are also present in a variety of tissues, including the autonomic nervous system, and the neuromuscular junction. The presence of these receptor sites throughout our bodies helps explain why some snake bites are so deadly. The venom that snakes release enters our bodies and quickly binds to nicotinic receptor sites, blocking cellular activity and causing paralysis. Antivenin is an antibody that seeks out and also binds to the toxic protein in the venom, hence protecting receptor sites from blockage.

Though snake bites can be lethal, humans have learned to similarly manipulate nicotinic receptors to their advantage. Some analgesics, known colloquially as "painkillers," work by binding to nicotinic receptors, relieving us from the experience of pain.

riety of pharmaceutical companies, trying to understand, develop, and assess various other compounds that would safely stimulate nicotinic receptors without encouraging addiction. While I was at Johns Hopkins in the 1980s, one of the first drug studies I ever conducted in Alzheimer's disease was with Nicorette chewing gum, an early smoking-cessation product that includes nicotine as its active ingredient. However, it was difficult to get patients to chew enough gum (which tasted terrible) and to be sure that they got adequate levels of nicotine in this way. The study was not a huge success, but some pharmaceutical companies did take our nicotinic research seriously and sought to adapt their own approaches.

In the 1990s, I visited the huge National Japanese Tobacco Institute, which has a pharmaceutical division. I also became a member of the highest-level consulting group to Abbott Pharmaceuticals. Abbott had developed a compound called ABT-418 that was bound to nicotinic receptors and administered to patients with Alzheimer's disease using a skin patch. There was some early evidence that these patients benefited on memory tasks, but for safety and other reasons the compound was not developed further.

In the late 1990s, I worked with Professor Jerry Yesavage and his team at Stanford University on a blinded randomized controlled trial that assessed donepezil (he also studied nicotine and other drugs) in pilots, of whom the average age was fifty-three. Rather than observe actual flying behavior, we studied these pilots in a flight simulator. Under these conditions Jerry could simulate emergencies and other challenges. Remarkably, but perhaps not terribly surprisingly since we all lose some cholinergic cells as we age, those pilots who received the cholinesterase inhibitor rather than a placebo landed better under difficult conditions and handled emergencies better.[4] Studies such as this suggest that there is a role for cholinomimetic drugs in enhancing cognition, not only for those who are elderly, but also for other people, perhaps even those younger than middle age, who are confronting challenging situations.

Some theorize that beyond cognitive enhancement, nicotinic drugs might even prevent age-related brain damage. Researchers, including my friend Professor Shun Shimohama in Kyoto, Japan, have conducted experiments in which nicotine is added to petri dishes containing nerve cells and various toxic substances present in the brain that are thought to kill neurons, such as beta-amyloid protein and excitatory amino acids such as glutamate. Remarkably, nicotine appears to minimize cell damage and provide a protective effect. Epidemiology studies have indicated that this protective effect may have some credence in human populations, since smokers have often been shown to have lower rates of neurodegenerative diseases such as Parkinson's. Some early studies suggested a "protective" effect for Alzheimer's, but later and better-designed studies showed the opposite: more dementia with more smoking.[5]

Ultimately, while I do hold some hope for drugs acting on nicotinic receptors, I must stress that the potential of these compounds is limited. Eventually, cholinergic drugs may provide some better ability to improve symptoms, but large effects associated with disease modification are less likely in my opinion. *I must also reiterate that readers should not start smoking or chewing nicotine gum to receive a cognitive enhancement! The small boost smokers receive pales in comparison to the drastic health risks that accompany each inhalation of carcinogen-laced smoke.*

CHOOSING PILLS OR NOT

I'm sure many of you are wondering how exactly you should navigate a treatment route of drugs and whether other pills and herbs can provide similar benefits at a lesser monetary cost and with lower risk of side effects. Because I was a contributor to the development of cholinesterase inhibitors, it is disappointing for me to see that treatments just haven't worked as we hoped they would. We have FDA-approved pills, but they don't contribute enough to quality of life to justify using them with my patients across the board. I have come to this conclusion: *It is more important to de-emphasize the role of medications in caring for brain aging and focus on other forms of non-medical, humanistic interventions to promote quality of life.* This is ultimately a judgment call a family unit has to make. For some people cholinesterase inhibitors show some benefit, and for others the effects are nonexistent or harmful. In practice, many of the positive effects that we see are probably related to placebo effects—and placebos are cheaper!

Gary Naglie, a geriatrician in Canada, recently reviewed the entire corpus of drug studies of ChEIs and found only four of ninety studies in which quality of life was even assessed directly. No positive results were found. However, it *is* becoming clear that some psychosocial interventions improve quality of life, for example, exercise programs and training community-based care coordinators.[6] Again, it must be emphasized that humans are adapted to receive care from one another and not exclusively from pills alone. Our treatment regimens should reflect this reality.

QUALITY OF LIFE AND HOW THE PHARMACEUTICAL INDUSTRY CAN HELP

In November of 2006, we held an international conference in Cleveland entitled "Reflecting on 100 Years of Alzheimer's Disease: The Global Impact on Quality of Lives." Indeed, achieving better quality of life for our elders—rather than producing a cure—was a main theme throughout the two-day event, which was attended by people from several national and international drug companies.

> I was particularly pleased that the Japanese company Eisai was represented by a senior official at the event. Eisai developed donepezil, and their corporate motto is "HHC" (human health care). Accordingly, they have supported many psychosocially oriented programs to complement their innovative biological efforts, which is commendable.

Naturally, one might ask how the pharmaceutical industry can improve its commitment to and measurement of quality of life in the future? One answer to this is narrative. Taking the vast collage of our experiences, emotions, and physical, mental, and spiritual states and synthesizing them into a cumulative "quality of life" requires us to tell detailed stories about ourselves. If clinical researchers and drug companies are truly interested in what role pharmacological interventions play in improving people's well-being, they must attune themselves to the experiential stories of the consumers who use pharmacological products.

We have at our disposal right now a tool that can facilitate the exchange of personalized narrative and quality of life information: the Internet.

THE INTERNET

There are already organizations such as Dementia Advocacy and Support Network International (DASNI) that provide space for online chat rooms for persons affected by dementia. Visit their site at www.dasninternational.org.

In the future, evaluation projects might reach out to their consumers by offering online blogging spaces that enable consumers to detail their experiences with drugs. Content analysis could be performed by computers to search for common words and themes that might elucidate broader conclusions about the quality of life conferred by particular drugs. One could imagine the drug companies might play a role in this process, although the ethical issues would be considerable.

If it could be worked out, such an assessment of future drug efficacy can be both intensely *personal,* in that drug companies would engage customers on the most intimate of terms, and *overarching*, in that tracking individual stories may be a reflection of larger consumer patterns that can then help drug companies sell more, and, most important, more effective, drugs. Needless to say, the drug companies that pay the most attention to the words and stories of their individual customers and adapt their product to suit consumer demands will gain a distinct competitive advantage over other companies. This should be the *real* meaning of personalized medicine.

The benefits of a comprehensive online quality of life measure won't pay dividends for drug company stockholders alone. By creating space for the sharing of stories, the Internet also empowers consumers to voice their opinions and join in protest against ineffectual drugs. These amplified voices give the pharmaceutical industry incentives to stay permanently attuned to their clients' subjective experiences with drugs, and to keep bringing innovative treatments to the market that will enhance quality of life. The stranglehold that drug companies now have over consumers would be loosened and large numbers of patients and caregivers could be mobilized against the complacency and false boasts of a pharmaceutical industry that is slow to innovate products such as ChEIs, but quick to market them to consumers and doctors.

EVALUATING "BREAKTHROUGHS"

In the June 18, 1990, issue of *Time*, a headline proclaimed, NEW HOPE FOR ALZHEIMER'S VICTIMS. The article reported that "it will soon be easier to identify Alzheimer's earlier and more accurately," and added that "Alzheimer's appears to be yielding to treatment." Since both predictions have failed to come true during the last two decades, the article teaches us a vital lesson: *We must learn to read media reports carefully so that we are not seduced by false hope.*

EVALUATING "BREAKTHROUGHS" THAT MAKE HEADLINES

Epidemiological studies have suggested that the use of nonsteroidal anti-inflammatory drugs (NSAIDs), including ibuprofen, naproxen, and indomethacin, may reduce the risk of AD, but clinical trials on human beings have not demonstrated a benefit. In fact, NSAIDs have been shown to cause gastrointestinal bleeding, as well as liver and kidney toxicity, which have limited their usage with the elderly.

Similarly, another popular news story has been that estrogen therapies will protect the brain and slow Alzheimer's. Again, most clinical trials have found that using estrogen to treat AD is not effective, and a link has been established between estrogen therapy and breast cancer. A large study found that women who took estrogen alone or with a synthetic progestin were actually at increased risk of developing dementia.

Another possibility is that taking statins—drugs normally prescribed to help manage cholesterol—will lower AD risk. Several human trials are under way but have not so far demonstrated a consistent positive effect. Statins can, however, cause serious muscle damage.

There are scores of medical stories in all forms of media that indicate a breakthrough is right around the corner. The overexaggerated promises made in headlines and on the evening news may be grandiose and comforting, but we must read with caution and learn to analyze these promises by sifting out the pertinent information from the pabulum. Here are a few tips to protect against false hope:

Use your head when reading the headline

The first lesson is to guard against being misled by sensationalistic headlines. If something sounds too good to be true, it probably is. Second, readers should take care to look beyond the facile language in headlines and into the body of the text where qualifiers are often used to describe the breakthrough. For instance, in the 2005 summer issue of *Newsweek*, an article called "7 Ways to Save a Brain" alleged that while "current treatments don't slow the underlying disease process . . . researchers are now testing an array of new therapies *intended* to do just that." It also reports that "better treatments *could* help patients . . . stay out of nursing homes" and that "these are *becoming* real possibilities." These important qualifiers that I have italicized are easy to miss when tantalizing headlines imply cures for Alzheimer's disease and play to our desire for hope. But words such as those in this article alter its meaning and belie the unrealistic hope for salvation from brain aging suggested by the headline.

Know the background of those claiming the "breakthrough"

As you are reading such stories, pay close attention to the sources and gauge whether the news agency can be trusted to have done accurate reporting or whether it has a reputation for sensationalism. Knowing the backgrounds of the experts quoted is also important. Remember that researchers have their careers and their funding bound up in the work they are doing and are not likely to give modest assessments of their progress. One of the biggest mistakes made by the two characters in *Waiting for Godot* was to place their abiding trust in a man whose motives they knew nothing about. Don't make the same mistake. Always strive to know as much as you can about the people who are making promises to you.

Of mice and men: Evaluate animal models

Another telling factor is how an article describes the evidence for the benefit of the medication. Is it an animal study, an epidemiological population study, or a randomized control trial on human beings? In many studies, compounds are tested on animals—most commonly mice—that have been genetically modified to overproduce the beta-amyloid protein seen in AD. The problem with these studies is that animal models are insufficient to study human maladies because a mouse brain is far less complex than a human brain, and since transgenic animals only mimic a high burden of BAP (and sometimes, but not always, neurofibrillary tangles), they constitute an insufficient frame of reference for human beings. On the basis of this discrepancy, and because of the wide anatomical gap between mice and men, you must take the best-laid plans you read in newspaper articles with a grain of salt.

Don't be seduced by simple solutions

Quite often, stories will purport that epidemiological evidence has shown that certain treatments or diets or lifestyles seem to lower prevalence rates in particular geographical, ethnic, or gender populations. Such studies can be encouraging, but usually do not prove anything definitively or display significant enough results to shift our practice. Population studies often miss out on individual variation and can be distorted by confounding factors even if attempts are made to correct for potential bias. For instance, the numbers seem to show that there is lower prevalence of dementia in some Indo-Asian cultures, and several researchers have attempted to draw a direct association between this low dementia incidence and variables such as diet. Diet is undoubtedly an important aspect of prevention, but there are innumerable other factors—for instance, genetic and socioeconomic factors—that contribute to brain aging, which confound the simplistic correlation of Indo-Asian diets, and any single component in those diets.

Look for the so-called gold standard of the randomized control trial

A scientific breakthrough for Alzheimer's disease that might affect practice would require randomized control trials (RCTs) that use human subjects and demonstrate that a treatment is efficacious over a placebo. In an RCT, consenting participants are randomly allocated into two or more groups, treatment groups and a control group. The former groups are given an experimental treatment, and the control group is given a placebo. The best-designed studies are so-called double-blind experiments. This means that throughout the duration of the trial, every participant and investigator in the study is unaware—or blind to—which group the person receiving treatment is in. Assigning patients into the two categories randomly and tracking their progress through time increases the probability that any measurable differences between the groups can be causally attributed to the treatment. Any study you come across that fails to do this should be approached with great caution and treated as exploratory and nothing more. Thus, scientists often refer to RCTs as the "gold standard" for research.

In the event that you encounter positive, scientifically sound RCT studies that seem to offer hope, you must still be cautious. The effect sizes are often small and exaggerated by the authors, especially in studies supported by the drug companies. In many cases, placebos cause improvements, and sometimes perform better than biologically active treatments. Furthermore, side effects are often underreported and studies are often not of long enough duration to establish long-term safety. Moreover, people who participate in RCTs are often carefully selected to be healthier or to have more clear-cut diagnostic categories. The result of this group biasing is that medications that are efficacious in these rarefied subgroups may not be effective in larger community-based samples where people may have co-morbidities (effects of additional disorders or diseases) or be less compliant in taking their medications.

Don't let hope become hype

Lastly, be aware of your own personal biases and tendencies in reading the story. We all have our interest piqued by headlines such as NEW HOPE FOR ALZHEIMER'S VICTIMS. Are you inclined to trust the information because it seems sound and logical, or because you want to believe it? Read with caution. A careful analysis of the surfeit of stories on AD can help you keep abreast of recent advances and maintain a sense of optimism without building up unrealistic expectations and false hope. The key is to read carefully, and keep your faith on a short leash.

CONTEMPLATING COMPLEMENTARY AND ALTERNATIVE TREATMENTS

For millennia, many people around the world have depended on so-called complementary and alternative medicines (CAMs) for their primary health care. In the West, the therapeutic market has undergone profound changes in the past decades, allowing Westerners to have more access to ancient nonconventional therapies. A wide range of alternative treatments, including diet, nutritional products, herbal supplements, and other interventions, are providing therapeutic options. CAM approaches are so entrenched that, in 2006, *The New York Times* reported that 48 percent of adults in America used at least one alternative or complementary therapy during 2004. Billions of dollars are spent each year out of pocket since medical insurance often does not cover these nonconventional approaches.

People are beginning to realize that the Western biomedical model neglects fundamental facets of the healing experience, namely, its narrative and relational aspects. When patients see the inadequacies of Western medicine up close—a misdiagnosis, a drug with negative side effects, botched surgery, even a dismissive doctor—many find the experience disillusioning.

Nonconventional approaches offer people the promise of personalized care, unhurried service, freedom from prescription drug side effects, and the potential for feeling not just physically better but also spiritually recharged.

Yet these treatments can also result in harm to the body and to the pocketbook and many are justifiably skeptical of CAM approaches because they lack the formal accountability of Western medicines. The best advice on selecting CAM treatments really comes down to being an educated consumer and knowing a treatment regimen and its provider well before participating in it.

Despite booming sales figures and mounting popularity in the West, CAM approaches are controversial because of concern about their efficacy, safety, and cost. Many Western doctors ignore and even ridicule alternative approaches because of the lack of systematic studies, particularly well-controlled randomized controlled trials that are the hallmark of drug development. Traditional therapeutic interventions are complex and highly subjective, and this makes it difficult to assess the nature of their effects. In the West, we tend to rely on objective data from RCTs, yet in most cases such data is not available for CAM approaches. Though healthy skepticism is necessary, outright dismissive stances toward CAM approaches are unreasonable. Doctors have a duty to be aware of what other means their patients are using to treat their symptoms and should be interested in what CAM approaches have to teach us about the many facets of healing, including the power of faith and spiritual beliefs.

INTEGRATING CAM INTO WESTERN CARE

Many, including myself, believe that CAM and Western scientific medicine can coexist. I tend to prefer the expression "integrative medicine" over CAM and for ten years directed an Office of Integrative Studies at Case Western Reserve University. In academic scholarship, integrative studies implies transdisciplinarity: a search for synthesis and not just reductive approaches. In health care, the word *integration* challenges all approaches to provide holistic care for patients. The traditional approaches of modern medicine form the foundation of our care, but we can build on the strengths of unconventional approaches, and build in the power of spirituality, which so many patients bring to the healing process. Scientific medicine tends to want to go to war with nature, whereas integrative approaches are more ecological and see human beings as a part of nature rather than somehow separate.

VISUAL THERAPY

I have friends in California named Bonnie and David Bell who create mandalas that are computer-generated collages composed of objects from nature that serve as a source of contemplation. Mandalas come in various forms—often round with symmetrical quadrants. The Bells' mandalas are complex images that resemble what one might see while looking through a kaleidoscope. Bonnie and David made me a personalized mandala I call "Deep Bioethics"; it is made largely from variegated rocks I have collected from around the world. Bonnie also created an image for her mother, who has some memory impairment, and joined it with soothing music, which together, help calm her mother's anxiety. It is more than conceivable to think that mandalas could potentially have therapeutic benefit, especially for those in the later stages of dementia who are more inclined to agitation. You can learn more about mandalas at www.gaiastarworld.com/index.html.

In my own practice, I am sympathetic to the general conceptions of health and healing evident in many integrative approaches. Non-Western medicine tends to be less microscopic, more ecological, more concerned about the influence of nature on human healing and the intricate relationships between elements that contribute to disease and suffering. Integrative medicines tend to focus on the responsibility of the patient in getting and staying well, and on prevention and maintenance of health rather than the exclusive treatment of disease. Many alternative traditions teach that health occurs in a community context. They emphasize the dynamic relationship among the individual, the healer, and the community as essential to a sense of connection and belonging that promotes the health of the individual and the community.

BEWARE OF HUCKSTERS

To persons coping with dementia, the U.S. Department of Health and Human Services offers this advice, which I quite agree with: "Because AD is such a devastating disease, caregivers and patients may be tempted by untried, unproven, unscientific cures, supplements, or prevention strategies. Before trying pills or anything else that promises to prevent AD, people should use caution and check with their doctor first. These purchases might be unsafe or a waste of money. They might even interfere with other medical treatments that have been prescribed."[7] You need not get rubber-stamp approval from your doctor on all health-related decisions you make, but if you have a good relationship with your doctor it's always good to ask.

Homeopathy

The premise of homeopathy is that minute amounts of active natural compounds, often the sources of synthetic medications produced by pharmaceutical companies, can be diluted into water to treat various problems. Homeopaths argue that the water retains the memory of the herb or mineral's vital essence, hence the healing power of the solution. Many critics express disbelief on the grounds that such diluted medicines could never have profound physiological effects, and that any positive outcome is surely due to the placebo effect. But part of the appeal of homeopathy is that its remedies are patient-centered and tailored to the individual. A homeopath will assess not just the physical cause of the illness but also the emotional state of the patient and her personality and temperament, before deciding what remedy or combination of compounds to use. As many of us in the healing profession know, basic empathy is a very powerful instrument of healing.

> The highest ideal of cure is the speedy, gentle, and enduring restoration of health by the most trustworthy and least harmful way.
>
> —SAMUEL HAHNEMANN,
> FOUNDER OF HOMEOPATHY

Homeopathy has been criticized on several fronts. For one, it has sometimes failed to demonstrate benefit in well-controlled studies. For example, in August 2005, the British medical journal *The Lancet* published a meta-analysis of eight trials of homeopathy selected from 110 placebo-controlled homoeopathy trials and 110 matched conventional medicine trials. The outcome of this meta-analysis suggested that the clinical effects of homeopathy are likely to be attributable to the placebo effect. The *Lancet* study does not prove that homeopathy is never effective or that all its accomplishments are rooted in the placebo effect, but it does raise major questions about the plausibility of homeopathy as a mainstream treatment.

My friend Kim Jobst is the editor of *The Journal of Alternative and Complementary Medicine,* as well as a homeopath himself, and I serve on his editorial advisory board. He and his colleagues strongly disagreed with the conclusions drawn by *The Lancet* and critiqued the journal on scientific and political grounds for publishing an error-filled, data-deficient study that "fail[ed] totally to provide the information necessary for full independent replication or analysis."[8]

THE POWER OF PLACEBOS

All healing traditions including Western medicine depend at least in part on the power of the placebo, which is an inert, biologically inactive substance used in drug trials to measure the incremental benefit of an active drug. The healing potential of placebos is evident, remarkable even in people with dementia who may not remember they are taking a pill. Many drugs have a tremendously difficult time showing that they have significant benefit over placebos, demanding that we give the placebo effect more clinical and scientific attention. Studies have consistently shown that the very act of going to see a doctor has therapeutic benefit, and that ongoing interaction with medical personnel can improve clinical outcome even when no biological treatment is involved.

Further criticism is leveled at the premises of homeopathy, which some say are inconsistent with the laws of chemistry. It is difficult to believe that a treatment would be made more powerful through a process of dilution, especially when no molecules of the original ingredients are present in the final treatment. In other words, those who seek homeopathic treatments are putting their faith in spiritlike therapeutic power that ostensibly defies our laws of science. My advice: Proceed with equal parts caution and open-mindedness if you elect to pursue homeopathic treatments.

Chiropractic

Unlike homeopathy, chiropractic treatment has made its way more successfully into the mainstream and has succeeded in achieving some degree of tolerance by Western medicine. The manipulation of the spine and various forms of massage have been demonstrated with fair consistency in some well-designed studies to have benefit in some conditions. Perhaps understandably, these approaches are most effective when dealing with musculoskeletal problems. At the very least, chiropractic treatments and massage can contribute to cognitive health by reducing anxiety and lowering stress. As you will see later, stress increases levels of certain hormones that may adversely affect the neuronal functioning of the hippocampus and other parts of the brain central to memory.

> *The nervous system holds the key to the body's incredible potential to heal itself.*
> —SIR JAY HOLDER, M.D., D.C., PH.D.,
> MIAMI, FLORIDA

Yoga and meditation

Yoga, tai chi, and meditation are centuries-old practices that train the mind and body to relax and appreciate each other by means of body postures, controlled breathing, and visualization exercises. Having practiced these forms from time to time, I can attest to their ability to contribute to relaxation and enhancement of mental well-being. Yoga and tai chi are low-impact and widely available, making them some of the safest and most accessible therapeutic options available to seniors. In addition to relaxation, yoga and meditation can promote mindfulness, allowing us to avoid distraction and maintain a sense of presence and coherence.

> *The best cure for the body is a quiet mind.*
> —NAPOLEON BONAPARTE

When you find a class that sounds interesting, it is not a bad idea to call ahead and ask whether the instructor has experience working with elderly persons. Also, it is wise to ask which classes are most suitable for beginners, and to check whether the instructor can make the necessary provisions for your mobility difficulties or cognitive needs. In fact, some instructors will have received training specifically for teaching aging persons. If taking classes is cost-prohibitive, consider searching for a video or audiotape on yoga for older audiences.

> *Dementia releases the essential self; we wander backward uncontrollably and become more of what we already were. But what I wonder is whether there is any way to train ourselves before we start to wander, so that when we lose our minds we are at peace. Yogis sit in caves for years. The rest of us have to earn a living. Serenity could be a forward-looking skill, though, if only we had time to acquire it.*
> —DR. ELISSA ELY, IN AN AUGUST 5, 2006,
> *NEW YORK TIMES* OP-ED PIECE

Acupuncture

Many years back, I remember being in a hospital in Beijing, China, and seeing a man diagnosed with multi-infarct dementia receiving acupuncture. What interested me most was how a traditional Eastern treatment was integrated with Western scientific medicine in a clinical setting like this. In China, separate medical schools train physicians in each tradition, but each school is well aware of and accepting of the other's approach. Whereas physicians being trained in Eastern medicine receive considerable training in modern scientific medicine, the allopathic physicians in China are much more aware and embracing of traditional approaches. Hence, it was acceptable for a man with scientifically diagnosed dementia to be receiving acupuncture treatment in a Western-style hospital. This is an integrative model America would be wise to learn from.

Various schools of acupuncture exist, each emphasizing different energy meridians—the force lines that are said to exist in the body, upon which different types of needles are placed. Dating back to the first century B.C., acupuncture is based on Asian medicine's sense of the flow of energy (qi, pronounced "chi") in the body and the need to maintain its balance.

*There is evidence that acupuncture influences the pro-
duction of and distribution of a great many neurotransmitters and neuromodulators.*

—David Eisenberg, M.D.,
Harvard Medical School

The practice teaches that disease is caused by a loss of homeostasis in
the body and that correcting one's flow of energy can restore wellness and
relieve pain. There are legitimate training programs and considerable empirical evidence that acupuncture appears to have effects beyond placebo,
particularly for the treatment of pain. Whether the therapy can directly increase a patient's verbal and motor skills, improve mood, memory, and
cognitive function, or increase endogenous levels of neurotransmitters as
has been claimed is another story. It is necessary to keep an open mind
about acupuncture and to assess its potential benefit in your life. If the
treatment intrigues you, it may be a worthy investment. Remember to do
your homework. Make sure that you ask for the qualifications of the prac-
titioner you are seeing, and do background research so that you know
what the treatment will entail and whether you will be comfortable undergoing it.

Herbs and naturopathy

Throughout the history of our species, humans have turned to the products
of nature to assist in healing. Modern scientific medicine depends on plants
and animals as a source of chemical substances that might hold therapeutic
benefit.

Ginkgo biloba. There is some evidence that ginkgo may have a positive effect on cognition and memory by promoting blood flow to the brain, but it
is not proven or approved by the FDA. The mechanism of action of ginkgo
is uncertain but it is thought by some to promote blood flow. As with many
herbals, it difficult to know the composition of the substances that you're
buying. *Consumer Reports,* for example, has identified that there is wide
variability in the amount of active ingredients in various ginkgo products
sold over-the-counter. Two companies in Europe developed a standardized
variant of ginkgo that has been used in many therapeutic trials. One of

those trials—a four-year randomized control trial on the effects of the herb—is currently being conducted at the University of Pittsburgh.

Ginseng. Widely used in Asia for its stimulant properties, although, as with ginkgo, ginseng's mechanism of action and therapeutic effects are not clear, ginseng is obtained from various plants from the *Panax* genus (provocatively translated as "all healing" in Latin), including some used by indigenous peoples in North America. There was a small spike in the popularity of ginseng after it was reported that rats fed high doses of the herb learned the layout of a maze quicker than rats in a control group. The theory was that ginseng acted as a cholinergic agent, increasing levels of acetylcholine in the brain. These findings were not consistently replicated, and since we lack data on the long-term safety of ginseng ingestion, it is difficult to recommend the herb clinically.

Fish oil and alpha lipoic acid. These compounds have been claimed to lower inflammation, cholesterol levels, and oxidative stress in animal models. Epidemiological data suggests that the consumption of foods high in omega-3 fatty acids may provide protection against Alzheimer's and other age-related conditions. Again, adequate human trials have not yet been performed, and fish oil, though in vogue, should not be seen as a panacea. Ultimately, it may be better to obtain your fish oils from real fish because you will also ingest vitamins and minerals that can help you metabolize the oil into its potentially neuroprotective components. However, one should be wary of high levels of mercury and other toxins found in some fish populations.

Huperzine A. This Chinese herb has shown some facility for improving memory in elderly people. Huperzine A is an alkaloid isolated from club moss that acts as a cholinesterase inhibitor. It has relatively few side effects and might eventually be proven to be efficacious in a fashion similar to other cholinesterase inhibitors. Studies are currently being done, and the jury is still out. I do not formally recommend this herb in my practice.

Galantamine. A phytonutrient, or plant-based nutrient, galantamine has a history of use that goes back at least 3,200 years. Galantamine is the active ingredient in the cholinesterase inhibitor Razadyne. Some scholars believe that in the Greek epic *The Odyssey*, galantamine, in the form of an extract from the snowdrop flower, was presented by Hermes to the hero, Odysseus, who used it as an antidote to protect himself from the goddess Circe's mind-altering drugs. Circe had used her potion to induce amnesia and a delusional state in Odysseus's crew. With the help of galantamine, Odysseus was able to retrieve the lost memories of his crew and protect his own memory, enabling them to continue their journey to their beloved homeland of Ithaca.

Folic acid and vitamins B$_{12}$ and B$_6$. Some studies have demonstrated that elevations in the level of an amino acid called homocysteine are associated with increased risk for stroke and a loss of cognitive performance characteristic of Alzheimer's disease. Folic acid and vitamins B$_{12}$ and B$_6$ are co-factors in homocysteine's metabolic pathways, and their presence in the body may potentially lower levels of this substance. This has prompted some physicians to recommend the three vitamins as supplements. Proof is lacking in the form of randomized controlled trials, although a recently published study appears to have confirmed the effect of folic acid supplementation on cognitive performance in human beings. Jane Durga et al. structured a randomized, double-blind, placebo-controlled study that took place between November 1999 and December 2004 in the Netherlands. Researchers randomly assigned 818 male and female participants aged fifty to seventy 800 milligrams daily oral folic acid or placebo for three years. The effect on cognitive performance was measured as the difference between the two groups in the three-year change in performance for memory, sensorimotor speed, complex speed, information processing speed, and word fluency. After three years, researchers noted that the changes in memory, sensorimotor speed, and information processing were significantly better in the folic acid group than in the placebo group.[9]

While these and other studies require replication before wholesale endorsement, some would argue that taking folate is harmless, and although the efficacy is not established, at least safety concerns are low.

Dehydroepiandrosterone (DHEA). A natural steroid hormone that is a precursor for androstenedione, testosterone, and estrogen, DHEA is sold as an oral supplement to improve memory, mood, and other endocrine functions. Because of its association with the sex hormones, particularly estrogen, it was thought perhaps to have an effect on cognition. However, a recent review by the Cochrane Collaboration—an evidence-based healthcare database centered in Oxford, England—demonstrated no consistent positive benefits in several studies.

IF IN DOUBT, ASK ARCHIE

The Cochrane Collaboration is the largest international effort to evaluate medical evidence and provide information to decision makers concerned about the quality of care in medicine. It was started by the British medical researcher Archie Cochrane in 1993. You can access this database at www.cochrane.org/index.htm. The Cochrane Library includes reviews of drugs, herbals, CAM, and other health-care interventions.

Hydergine. When I started my practice, the only drug available to treat people with Alzheimer's disease was hydergine. It was not actually approved for Alzheimer's but rather for symptoms of cognitive insufficiency in older adults. It was made by a drug company in Switzerland called Sandoz, which has now merged with other companies.

Hydergine was widely promoted and was once one of the best-selling medicines in the world. Its mechanism of action was unclear: It was first seen as a vasodilator, as were many early drugs when it was felt that an insufficient blood supply to the brain was the cause of dementia. It then became known as a cerebral metabolic enhancer, and finally was said to affect cholinergic mechanisms. In other words, the mechanism of its action tended to mimic the current theory of the cause of dementia that was in vogue at the time. There was actually some evidence in randomized control trials that it had modest effects on a rather vague profile of dementia symptoms, including impaired cognition. However, hydergine was approved by the FDA before modern standards for efficacy were introduced. With the advent of the modern drugs such as the cholinesterase inhibitors mentioned earlier in the chapter, hydergine sales have slipped. However, the medicine is still sold in various countries around the world and I would not dissuade my patients from taking it.

Piracetam. Another drug that was introduced early on to treat cognitive problems in the elderly was piracetam, produced by a company in Belgium. A Google search will indicate an almost miraculous number of conditions that can be treated with the substance. Once again, its mechanism of action is unclear but it is purported to be a cerebral metabolic enhancer. As with hydergine, there are studies that show that it may have a positive effect on some cognitive symptoms in some patients. The Cochrane Review confirms that evidence is suggestive of positive effects but calls for renewed research rather than current clinical use.

AN INTERVENTION YOU NEEDN'T SWALLOW: VOLUNTEERING AT THE INTERGENERATIONAL SCHOOL

Not all treatments for dementia are medicinal in their nature. In my hometown of Cleveland, Ohio, my wife, Cathy, and I, along with numerous friends and colleagues, have developed a community-based initiative: the world's first intergenerational charter school (www.tisonline.org). In existence for five years, The Intergenerational School (TIS) has received international recognition as well as state, regional, and local awards for its educational excellence. It is committed to innovation in public education, with a pedagogical focus on lifelong, developmentally appropriate learning in service of community.

> *What is my life if I am no longer useful to others?*
> —JOHANN WOLFGANG VON GOETHE

Children aged six to twelve celebrate learning in the company of older adults. Some of these older adults are students from local colleges (including my university, Case Western Reserve); others are senior citizens with memory challenges, some of whom have received Alzheimer's diagnoses and pills for their condition. One such volunteer is Mrs. Mary Atwood, a Cleveland resident who has been volunteering as a reading mentor for the last four years. Mrs. Atwood received a diagnosis of AD nearly five years ago. Ever since, she—AD label and all—has been one of our most steady volunteers and has helped dozens of children learn how to read. She has told my research assistants that, in her opinion, the weekly reading sessions she has with the children do more for her health and well-being than any prescription given to her. She relishes the opportunity to give back to her community and work with children—especially since her AD label can sometimes limit the relationships she can have with people. Visiting the school on Thursdays is the highlight of her week.

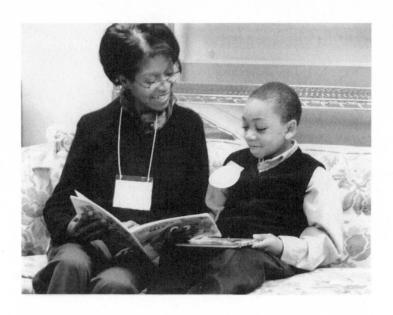

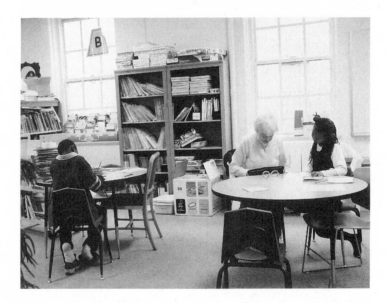

Figure 9. Reading and Mentoring.   The signature activity of TIS is the reading mentoring program. It is through books that children and elders can use their imaginations together to share stories with one another, as well as stories of their own lives (top photo). Many of our initial private foundation grants were used to create a rich library of children's literature, including carefully selected books that feature and foster intergenerational relationships. Featured in the second photograph is Mrs. Mary Atwood, a long-standing volunteer of the school and a patient in our clinic who has memory problems and a family history of early-onset dementia. She comes from a family of educators committed to teaching children important lessons of life, for example, concerning diversity. (Photos courtesy of Peter Whitehouse)

FINDING A PLACE TO VOLUNTEER

Obviously there is not yet an intergenerational school in every community. However, I would urge you to explore volunteer opportunities in your community, and to ask elementary schools in your neighborhood if they have reading programs or if they would consider developing them. Other organizations in your community you might approach for volunteer opportunities:

- local churches or faith-based groups

- local charities

- city hall and community affairs representatives

Should you be unsuccessful in your own community . . .

In the late 1990s an initiative called Civic Ventures was founded by John Gardner and my friend and colleague Marc Freedman. Civic Ventures is an organization that is reframing the debate about aging in America and redefining the second half of life as a source of social and individual renewal. Through programs and consulting, Civic Ventures brings together older adults with a passion for service and helps stimulate opportunities for using their talents to advance the greater good. Its program portfolio includes:

Experience Corps, a national service program for Americans over fifty-five. The program now operates in fourteen cities and links volunteers over age fifty-five with tutoring and mentorship opportunities in after-school programs. Learn more at www.experiencecorps.org/index.cfm.

The Next Chapter, an initiative that provides expertise and assistance to community groups across the country working to help people in the second half of life set a course, connect with peers, and find pathways to significant service.

The Lead with Experience Campaign and the Purpose Prize, a three-year initiative to invest in older social innovators by recognizing outstanding achievements, creating a network of people wanting to use their retirement years for the greater good, and channeling funds and assistance to these new pioneers.

The MetLife Foundation/Civic Ventures Breakthrough Award, for innovative organizations that tap the passion and experience of people over fifty to improve society.

For more info, visit www.civicventures.org.

In addition to reading, our other intergenerational programs focus on the use of computers, gardening, and other activities designed to stimulate the bodies and minds of learners of all ages and create opportunities for the mutual transfer of knowledge and wisdom. Gardening allows learners of all ages to learn about natural cycles, food production, and the enjoyment of natural settings. In The Intergenerational School, we are demonstrating that a different model of public education can not only provide better learning for children, but can also create opportunities for older adults to contribute in a purposeful way to the future of their communities, share their collective wisdom, and stay cognitively vital in the process.

This pedagogical model could also be implemented in different learning environments, for instance, in private schools and universities, as well as long-term-care facilities—volunteering can be more cognitively enhancing than any pill an older person can put in their body. Establishing spaces like the Intergenerational School will be vital for a society that will have so many aging persons with so much to give back.

When Cathy and I visited Finland, a country renowned for its public education system, they were most interested in our Intergenerational School because they believe that they have a cultural problem with "silent knowledge." This is the wisdom of elders that is going unheard by the younger generations because of changes in living patterns (families and their children are now living in separate locations from their grandparents). The recognition of this wisdom is a valuable lesson for American culture, and the rest of the aging world. Even with the limitations of old age we have much to learn from our elders. As Ernest Hemingway's venerable fisherman imparts to his young companion in *The Old Man and the Sea*, "I may not be as strong as I think . . . but I know many tricks and I have resolution."

It's safe to say, looking back over the past few decades of drug development, that the symptomatic therapies in Alzheimer's disease have failed to deliver the silver bullet that we've been waiting for. All of the cholinesterase inhibitors have an efficacy profile of modest at best, and their impact on the activities of daily living is minimal. The drug industry has not taken up the challenge of trying to determine whether these drugs really improve the quality of life of consumers. When clinicians deliberate over which pills to use, the decision usually has more to do with which pill has the least harmful side effects than which is the most effective. Dr. John Abramson put it well in his book *Overdosed America*: "Something is very wrong," he wrote, "with a system that leads patients to demand and doctors to prescribe a drug that provides no better relief and causes significantly more side effects."[10]

I've come a long way in my thinking about AD drugs. It wasn't that long ago that I was (legally) obtaining memantine and other medicines from Europe before they were approved in the United States. I wanted to believe in those approaches, but now I find it increasingly difficult to subject my patients to their limited benefits and potential side effects. Hundreds of thousands of elderly people are putting marginally effective pills into their bodies and suffering adverse side effects for small net gains. When the price of these pills—on average four dollars a day—is considered along with their pitfalls, we as a society must consider if marginal benefits justify high personal and societal costs. In my opinion, the future treatments for brain aging must be integrative. We must begin to move beyond the conventional therapies that have not delivered on their promise.

Quality of life can be improved, not by waiting for Godot, but by staying mentally and physically active and addressing the range of ecological factors that influence our cognitive health, which you will learn about in Part Three. Having a sense of purpose in life and a sense of belonging to a family and community is also critical to individual well-being. If physicians spend all their time talking about drugs, there is little time to discuss other life options that may contribute to preserving and even enhancing quality of life.

CHAPTER SIX

A Brave New World of Genetics and Molecular Medicine?[1]

I think it's safe to say we will have individualized, preventative medical care based on our own predicted risk of disease as assessed by looking at our DNA. By then each of us will have had our genomes sequenced because it will cost less than $100 to do that. And this information will be part of our medical record. Because we will still get sick, we'll still need drugs, but these will be tailored to our individual needs. They'll be based on a new breed of designer drugs with very high efficacy and very low toxicity, many of them predicted by computer models.

—Francis Collins, Director, National Human Genome Research Institute

In the year 2000 scientists completed the first survey of the human genome. Then-President Bill Clinton announced the accomplishment at a White House press conference, congratulating scientists working in the public and private sectors on what was a "landmark achievement, which promises to lead to a new era of molecular medicine, an era that will bring new ways to prevent, diagnose, treat, and cure disease."[1]

A new era had begun for the Alzheimer's field. Whereas yesterday's hope for AD was placed in understanding the systems of neurotransmitters in the brain, the new century brought a new hope for future tests and AD therapies based on molecular genetics and biology. My own career was involved in this transition from the systems neuroscience described in the previous chapter to the molecular age. Systems approaches had produced cholinesterase inhibitors, which ultimately did not achieve the level of clinical benefit for which we had hoped. Molecular approaches aggressively displaced systems neuroscience, becoming the dominant research approach and promising to delve more deeply into the basic question of why brain cells live and die. Copious funding began to pour in for molecular researchers who aimed to develop treatments that could preempt the first signs of disease-related damage in the brain rather than treat secondary symptoms as cholinesterase inhibitors did. Although I moved away from direct laboratory work as this evolution was taking place in the 1980s and 1990s, I hired several molecular scientists in my organization and have stayed connected to the molecular "march of progress."

As Francis Collins's quote at the beginning of the chapter suggests, the molecular medicine paradigm has promised to spawn an era of personalized medicine—a new age in which information about your genetic makeup may be used to tailor individual strategies for the detection, treatment, or prevention of disease. This seductive movement is predicated on three premises:

1. That we will be able to identify key genetic lesions associated with a particular disease or disease subgroup.

2. That we will have a variety of available treatments for particular diseases.

3. That we will be able to identify those genetic markers in such a way that we personally match the treatment with the individual. (This has led to the emergence of a field called pharmacogenomics, which, as the word implies, combines genetics with pharmaceutical treatments.)

According to personalized medicine, conditions like Alzheimer's disease are influenced by several genetic factors, and once we know the proper molecular markers, we can offer early diagnosis and prepare personalized treatments. Just how helpful the genetic paradigm can be for a condition such as Alzheimer's disease, which is clearly influenced by a variety of environmental and lifestyle factors, remains to be seen.

GENETICS 101

Genes are basic units of heredity that are located at specific points along the chromosomes in the nucleus of each cell in our bodies. They are, in essence, sequences of chemical units called nucleotides (abbreviated A, C, T, G) arranged in double-helix coils that provide coded instructions that lead to the expression of all of our characteristics. Genes have alleles—or alternative forms—that arise through mutation, contributing to the hereditary variation we see in human populations.

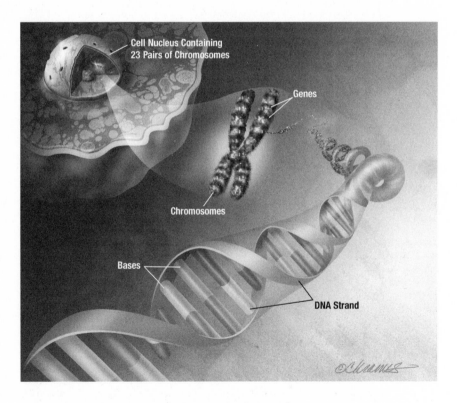

Figure 10. A Closer Look at DNA.   Our genetic material is located inside the nucleus of cells in structures called chromosomes. Chromosomes themselves are made up of DNA (and other substances); DNA is built from pairs of amino acid bases. (Courtesy of the National Institute on Aging, *Alzheimer's Disease: Unraveling the Mystery*)

THE GENETICS OF AD

In 1996 nearly 150 years after Gregor Mendel's groundbreaking theories on the hereditary properties of pea plants, a team of scientists led by Alan Roses of Duke University identified a susceptibility gene that might contribute to late-onset AD: the ApolipoporoteinE (ApoE) gene variant located on chromosome 19. Roses and his team hypothesized that this gene interacted with beta-amyloid to increase the risk of late-onset AD. As I mentioned in Chapter 2, the ApoE gene, which had previously been implicated as a genetic risk factor for heart disease, has three alleles (E2, E3, E4) that are unequally distributed in human populations throughout the world. Roses's group identified that individuals with two ApoE-4 alleles, one inherited from the mother and one inherited from the father, were more at risk for AD than those with other combinations of alleles, or those with only one copy of ApoE-4. They found that the ApoE-3 variant conferred an intermediate risk, while those with the ApoE-2 form appeared to have a lower risk. With regards to ApoE-4, about 35 to 50 percent of all people with so-called late-onset Alzheimer's have been found to have least one copy of the gene, compared to 25 percent in the general unaffected population.[2]

Unlike the autosomal dominant genes on chromosomes 1, 14, and 21 that are known to inevitably *cause* early-onset AD symptoms from ages thirty to fifty, susceptibility genes like ApoE-4 only *increase* risk. The presence of such genes as this does not mean that you will necessarily develop the condition in your later decades. An ApoE-4 allele may subject you to a greater susceptibility, but its presence does not cause the disease, nor does its absence protect you against the disease. You can die in your nineties with two copies of the ApoE-4 allele and not suffer severe cognitive impairment. Or you can be a carrier of two ApoE-2 alleles and become demented in your seventies. *In short: The ApoE alleles do not determine with certainty whether or not a person will develop AD. ApoE-4 is not a genetic time bomb.*

The search for so-called AD genes is altogether problematic in a complex condition such as brain aging, which is influenced by multiple developmental factors throughout life, and not merely one's genes. You can imagine one's genetic endowment as a blank canvas upon which the colors, textures, and shapes of one's life are thrown. The canvas is of course essential to the whole picture, but the process by which the picture is constructed is what is most compelling. Nevertheless, the reductionistic hunt for other inheritable susceptibility alleles that contribute to AD incidence continues. In 2001 a new potential gene site was identified on chromosome 10. Other sites currently under investigation are located on chromosomes 9, 12, 13, 15, and 19. Scientists frequently report that they have identified a new susceptibility gene, but many of these reports arouse considerable controversy.

APOE

As my colleagues Margaret Lock, Stephanie Lloyd, and Janalyn Prest have written, the concept of ApoE-4 is complex: "ApoE-4 has been shown to work in unexpected ways in certain populations. For instance, among Pygmies, and other populations whose subsistence economy was relatively recently predominantly that of hunting and gathering, ApoE-4 apparently protects against AD."[3] We have also recently learned that ApoE-4 may be protective against macular degeneration, a common cause of blindness in the elderly.[4]

GETTING TESTED FOR APOE

In recent years, some clinics have begun offering a test for people with memory problems to see if they are carriers of ApoE-4 as part of the diagnostic evaluation. Since the E-4 allele is associated with risk for other dementias besides Alzheimer's disease, it is not very helpful in narrowing down the diagnostic choices. The procedure has drawn much scrutiny, and all respected clinical guidelines from professional organizations recommend against the use of the ApoE test.

The most challenging ethical problem with ApoE testing involves whether clinicians should provide susceptibility risk information to asymptomatic individuals, given the imprecision of the information and the lack of any available treatment. Contrast that with a condition such as Phenylketonuria (PKU), a genetic disorder leading to neural defects that occurs in nearly one in fifteen thousand births. We have identified a deterministic gene for PKU—meaning that if you are a carrier of it you will express PKU symptomology—and we know that early intervention can lead to an effective treatment (a special diet low in phenylalanine) that enables affected persons to grow up with normal brains. The case is much different for ApoE-4, since it is not a deterministic gene, and since we lack effective treatments for persons who may be carrying the gene. Interestingly, even the company that markets the ApoE clinical test insists that it should not be used as a predictive test for people who do not have symptoms.

MY EXPERIENCE IN GENETIC COUNSELING

For the past six years, I have been funded by the National Human Genome Research Institute through its Ethical, Legal and Social Implications program (ELSI) and the National Institute on Aging study providing ApoE information to persons at risk for dementia. This work has been conducted with Melissa Butson in Cleveland, and with colleagues at Boston University (where my friend Bob Green is the overall study principal investigator), the University of Michigan, Cornell University, and Howard University.

During these six years, we have provided counseling to adult children and siblings of people with dementia for genetic-based risk assessment for AD using the ApoE gene. What we have been asking is whether people find ApoE testing information useful or stressful, or both. In short, individuals value the interaction with genetic counselors and appreciate the opportunity to obtain the latest genetic information. Though our participants have expressed ample amounts of confusion about the information, they did not become excessively depressed, nor did they commit suicide or take any other drastic action as a result of learning their genetic profile. Some bought long-term-care insurance. In general, we found that people do not fully recall or understand the genetic information they are given, and it is not clear that the actual information had a great deal of impact on their lives. Some of my collaborators feel more strongly that we are on the march to progress and that this kind of genetic information can be provided quickly and easily and help people plan their lives. I am not so optimistic about genetic advances clearly and easily improving quality of life.

Arguments in favor of genetic research are often based on the notion that the information received will fundamentally alter the decisions a person makes. But think about it in the context of your own life: Do you need genetic information to eat healthier, exercise, and take care of yourself; to be nicer to loved ones; to inspire you to volunteer in your community; to provide the impetus to pursue goals that you've not gotten around to, or to read a book like this? These and other life changes can be accomplished without an expensive genetic test that offers nebulous information. In the long run, it may be better to pay attention to your family history more than a genetic test, since many people intuit that they have a genetic risk merely by knowing about the fates of their relatives. Certainly, my fellow clinicians should use strong means of professional persuasion to convince their patients to act preventively—of course, this encouragement must be based on accurate and valid information.

GENETICS AND PROFIT

Many companies are beginning to market genetic tests that make extravagant claims about their ability to predict various dietary and therapeutic avenues. In April 2006, GenSpec Labs put out a line of vitamins that purportedly addresses the needs of different races. These "targeted-nutrient" pills, as they are called, contain elevated vitamin D and zinc and are aimed at African-Americans and Hispanics—populations said to be genetically predisposed to deficiencies in those nutrients. While the company defended their race-specific vitamins by invoking the notion that gender- and age-specific products are accepted in most developed economies, they were assailed on the basis that their product tacitly reinforces racial/ethnic divisions in society and reifies a genetic homogeneity that simply does not exist. As ABC News correspondent Dr. David Katz said, genetic reductionism is specious and unhelpful: "We make a mistake thinking we're all that different from each other. The differences in our health are more related to lifestyle, education, finances, and poverty than they are to genetics."[5]

THE DEPERSONALIZATION OF PERSONAL MEDICINE

I've always wondered if molecular-genetic medicine, which promises to foretell the details of a person's life and death, *de*personalizes and stresses individuals rather than enhances their wellness. Giving patients complex and ambiguous information about the risk of gene variants such as ApoE for which there is no known course of treatment can cause undue worry and may lead to unnecessary or harmful medical interventions. Reducing a person to her molecular-genetic profile seems a profoundly dehumanizing turn for modern medicine to take.

These misgivings have been confirmed by many of my patients, particularly one woman who came to see me for genetic consultation in neurology. While undergoing a preventive cardiology workup at another health-care institution, this woman had been identified as having genetic risk for cardiovascular disease (CVD). Her cardiologist mailed her results as a printout, which included the information that she expressed two copies of the E-4 allele of the ApoE gene, and that this phenotype had been found to be a susceptibility marker for CVD.

Concerned by her genetic profile, and unsure what all the jargon meant, the woman went to the library to conduct her own research. Through this she found out that she was not only at risk for cardiovascular disease, she was at more risk to develop Alzheimer's disease than those who have two of the more common ApoE-3 alleles.

The woman had already survived two bouts with cancer and felt that she had overcome her illnesses by taking a mind-over-matter approach. Quite understandably, she was terrified by the prospect that she might now lose her mind. She was infuriated that her genetic susceptibility for Alzheimer's had been so carelessly presented to her without any discussion of its broader implications in the context of her life, so much so that she considered filing a lawsuit against the cardiologist. I counseled her—as I do all who are concerned about their genetic risk for Alzheimer's disease— by emphasizing that the magnitude of risk is often difficult to assess. In contrast with the autosomal dominant genes on chromosomes 1, 14, and 21 that we know lead to early-onset dementia, normal brain aging is not fully determined by the family's genes. As you will learn more in Part Three, there are many environmental and lifestyle variables that contribute to the aging of our brains.

In a front-page article appearing on August 31, 2006, Gina Kolata of *The New York Times* nicely summarized the vacillating scientific view on the role of genetics in aging:

> The scientific view of what determines a life span or how a person ages has swung back and forth. First, a couple decades ago, the emphasis was on environment, eating right, exercising, getting good medical care. Then the view switched to genes, the idea that you either inherit the right combination of genes that will let you eat fatty steaks and smoke cigars and live to be a hundred or you do not. And the notion has stuck so that these days many people point to an ancestor or two who lived a long life and assume they have a genetic gift for longevity. But recent studies find that genes may not be so important in determining how long someone will live and whether a person will get some diseases—except, perhaps, in some exceptionally long-lived families. That means it is generally impossible to predict how long a person will live based on how long the person's relatives lived.

Indeed, genes are life's canvas, but experience is the series of brushstrokes upon that canvas that produce the compelling images that come to represent our embodied existence.

Having a parent or multiple relatives who are diagnosed with AD (clinically and pathologically) earlier in their lives clearly increases risk, but in a way that is difficult to quantify. My advice for my patient was that she should do her best to take care of her mind and body—the environmental and lifestyle factors over which she had control (eating well, exercising, keeping blood pressure and cholesterol low, and staying socially engaged)—and try not to dwell on the ambiguous genetic risk. In essence, that would be my advice to you, as well.

THE FALLACY OF RACE AND GENES

Human health is complex and holistic: No one variable in isolation can provide adequate causal explanation for disease patterns among ethnic groups. For more than fifty years there has been a persistent tendency to attribute health problems such as hypertension and AD amongst African-Americans to *intrinsic* African genes, despite extensive research that has clearly implicated *extrinsic* factors involving lifestyle, diet, and other ecological factors as being significant in increasing the differential risk. Efforts to link race, genes, and disease risk ultimately obscure significant environmental factors that are usually affected by socioeconomic inequality.

Because African-Americans are disproportionately represented in lower socioeconomic classes, they are more susceptible to suffering from the effects of poor nutrition, being exposed to neurotoxins such as mercury, lead, and arsenic in drinking water, acquiring less cumulative education relative to those in higher financial classes, holding less cognitively stimulating jobs, having less free time to exercise—all factors that have a bearing on brain health through the course of one's life. Genetic predisposition is only a small part of the story of a person's health.[6]

Had my patient's cardiologist taken the time to discuss the broad implications of that information, he would have told her that there was a considerable range of error around our estimates of susceptibility. This means that any ApoE risk assessment given to anyone must be taken as an imperfect approximation. For example, an ApoE-4 risk given at 35 percent might actually be 35 percent plus or minus 10 or even 15 percent. In other words, we would estimate the patient's risk of developing Alzheimer's-type dementia to be somewhere between 20 and 50 percent. These estimates vary because the population of people studied to generate our relative risk estimates is small, not representative of the general population, and the equations to calculate risk have fudge factors. We really do not know the full range of our possible error. As you can see, given the enormous range in our risk assessment, the integrity of our estimate breaks down, as does its potential usefulness to you or your loved ones.

> Several years ago, as part of the federal REVEAL project, I provided counseling to patients in Cleveland and confronted firsthand the confusion many have about genetics. One of my patients was an African-American woman who had two ApoE-4 alleles. This, along with the fact that she was African-American and a woman, meant that our data sets converged to give an extremely high AD risk of nearly 75 percent. I gave her countless caveats and qualifiers about the imperfections of our data sets. At the end of our counseling sessions, I felt comfortable that she recognized the limitations of the study, and that her equanimity was not unduly influenced by the risk calculation.

MORE LESSONS FROM MY PATIENT'S STORY

My patient's case demonstrates the multiple challenges our culture faces in moving genetic technology into the clinic. How can we expect people to react to concepts such as susceptibility and risk, particularly when this information is so vague and imprecise? How do we convert this knowledge into useful information? Larger questions arise about so-called personalized medicine. Do you want to be defined by your genes? Do you want your genetic blueprint to be the central narrative in your life, spelling out the relative risk for all your potential ailments? Is our health-care system prepared to assist individuals in adjusting their lives when they know something about their genetic predisposition to certain diseases?

Although mapping the human genome was certainly an awe-inspiring achievement for molecular biology and the discovery of the association between ApoE and AD a positive advancement in our understanding of the genetics of brain aging, none of our findings have resulted in clear advancements in the way we approach AD. Individual risk assessments are widely seen as being too vague to have any use in clinical care. The ethical questions these discoveries have engendered require us to pause to consider how we are going to manage this delicate information, how valuable it can really be to society at large, and whether we should choose to pursue it in our own lives.

GENETIC TREATMENTS FOR AD:
WHAT DOES THE FUTURE HOLD?

The discovery of the ApoE-AD link was an important development in the Alzheimer's field, insofar as it allowed us to make small advances in understanding its biology and genetics. Whether these baby steps were down the right path is what we now question, because the dominance of examining genetic mechanisms at work in Alzheimer's has necessarily limited other avenues of exploration into areas I would consider more profound—namely, the environmental and lifestyle factors that influence brain aging throughout one's life.

Beyond diagnostics, the most important implications for molecular-genetic research on Alzheimer's have more to do with treatment. Molecular medicine is being used as a platform to make new promises and pronouncements about curing Alzheimer's. The assumption now is that much more remains to be learned about the genetics of Alzheimer's and that with more knowledge we may make profound breakthroughs leading to medications. The AD empire has given us another reason to maintain our expectations for more powerful treatments such as amyloid vaccines, stem cells, and other pharmacogenetic innovations. It's *Waiting for Godot* all over again. None of our genetic findings have moved us closer to the prevention and/or treatment of Alzheimer's disease. Nevertheless, the purveyors of the AD myth continue to make big promises.

GETTING TO THE ROOT OF STEM CELLS

The biggest of those promises is stem cells, which have generated a good deal of attention and raised hopes and expectations for a cure. Stem cells are undifferentiated cells that retain the ability to divide and differentiate into other cell types. Their protean nature gives them the potential to act as a repair system for the body, in which they can be used to build specific tissues or grow organs through cellular therapy. The stem cell issue has become a political controversy: On one side are those who resist embryonic stem cell research on the ethical grounds that human embryos may be destroyed in order to derive certain populations of stem cells, and on the other side the scientific positivists who zealously support research contend that stem cell technology can be of limitless value, especially in conditions such as diabetes, cancer, spinal-cord injuries, and degenerative neurological conditions like Parkinson's and Alzheimer's. The national debate is usually waged along these polarized lines with little thought given to the scientific feasibility of stem cell treatments, especially in complex conditions such as AD, or to other ethical issues beyond the pro-life/pro-choice politicized issues. For example, we rarely consider the risks of injecting stem cells that have the potential for unlimited growth and could become a cancer.

The potential of stem cells is so great because they are pluripotent, that is to say, they are capable of affecting more than one organ or tissue. Stem cells from embryos seem to have particular flexibility, but undifferentiated cells can also be found in a variety of adult tissues as well as umbilical cord blood. Through human manipulation, both types of stem cells may potentially be grown into neurons and other specialized cells, enabling us to integrate them into targeted locations in the body where they might help regrow damaged cells in tissues and organ systems. This promises exciting opportunities for intervening in the progression of formerly incurable diseases and injuries, such as diabetes, paralysis, dementia, and other conditions in which unabated cell death causes human suffering. In fact, it is likely that stem cells will be more helpful in situations where one particular kind of cell is involved, as is the case in diabetes, where insulin-producing cells are located in the pancreas (although even in that relatively simple condition, experts say stem cell treatments are far away).

Excitement aside, the discourse on stem cells purveyed by politicians and the mainstream media is greatly oversimplified. Greed, exaggeration, and political expedience have prevailed over rational debate on the issue. It is my professional opinion, and the opinion of most real experts on the biology of AD and stem cells that I have talked to, that neither embryonic nor adult stem cells will prove to be as useful for Alzheimer's disease in both the near future and even the long term as some claim.

STEMMING THE TIDE: STRAIGHT TALK ON STEM CELLS

In an October 2005 talk entitled "Stem Cell Research: Hype or Hope," Dr. Austin Smith of Edinburgh, who directs EuroStemCell, a consortium for stem cell research, briefly discussed the ethical implications of current and future research. His closing remarks touched on the responsibility of scientists to tell the truth and not fuel false hope. He challenged the scientists on hand not to exaggerate the prospect for cures, not to underestimate research challenges, and not to trivialize issues of public anxiety with pseudoscience.

Directly after that, he took a few questions and my co-author was lucky enough to be called on. He pressed Smith more on the "hype vs. hope" theme, especially as it related to a multi-system neurological disorder such as Alzheimer's disease, and explained the dilemma we have when people ask us about the potential for a stem cell cure to AD. Smith responded by saying that he believed there was much "false hope" being propagated by politicians and journalists and that it was destructive to science and harmful to individuals who deserved to be told the truth. He also said that he had a hard time envisaging cell transplantation therapy for AD, and said it was much more plausible for the pharmaceutical industry to develop neuronal models based on stem cell research (to better understand degeneration). Leveling perspectives from leaders like Smith are much needed as we push forward in stem cell research. The grandiose promises made by scientists and pronounced at political conventions fuel false hope and set us up for potential disappointment.

Alzheimer's disease is a multi-system disorder that affects many brain regions. To recover function in memory, the implanted stem cells would have to form intricate connections with neurons in an older, diseased brain. This does not seem plausible. Nor have scientists explained just how growing new neurons will help us regain old memories.

A fixation on stem cell treatments may distract us from basic preventive measures that could contribute to arresting cell damage in the first place. All the energy put into stem cells could cause us to allocate our resources too narrowly, putting all our eggs in one basket, as the saying goes. Treating the multiple environmental and lifestyle factors that contribute to brain aging would be more effective than implanting stem cells in people's brains post-facto. As you will see in Chapter 9, minimizing damage to developing brains and maintaining a vigorous mental and physical life as we age can do more for individuals and communities than a biological fix.

Few credible scientific investigators in the Alzheimer's field believe that stem cells offer much future potential. For Parkinson's disease, the hope may be a bit more realistic. Although it also affects multiple neuronal populations, enhancing dopaminergic (dopamine-producing) cells does provide therapeutic benefit for some patients because this neurotransmitter, dopamine, seems to be important for bodily movement, which is disrupted in PD. However, many patients with Parkinson's become cognitively impaired later in the illness, suggesting that PD is also a multi-system condition that will resist easy answers. Implanted embryonic cells have already been tried in Parkinson's with mixed but not completely discouraging results.

A few leading researchers have had the courage to proclaim that we should stop waiting for Godot. Yet, excessive hype about curing these degenerative diseases and others has made stem cells an important political issue, with many applying intense pressure to commercialize stem cells. In 2003, California passed a constitution-modifying proposition called the "Stem Cells and Cures Act" that led to a $3 billion investment of public funds in stem cell research. The use of the word *cure* juxtaposed with *stem cells* is, in my view, irresponsible, since the phrase implies that positive outcomes will be had if the public simply invests its tax dollars in basic biological research. Human beings love simple answers for complex problems, and we are a great species because we often innovate and come up with answers. Unfortunately, the notion of using stem cells to ameliorate Alzheimer's disease is misleading and creates false hope.

HOPING FOR HOPE

While in Los Angeles several years ago, I heard Patti Davis, daughter of Ronald Reagan, attack the Bush administration for its opposition to stem cell research. Since people had pointed out to her that she might be articulating excessive hope for stem cells and AD, she insisted that there is no such thing as false hope. While I appreciated Patti's sentiment, I disagree. Creating high expectations and then dashing hope when the great weight of reality crashes down potentially creates more misery and suffering in the long run and is ethically and scientifically questionable.

NERVE GROWTH FACTOR (NGF) FIBROBLASTS

Another related therapeutic approach that is attracting considerable attention is the process of implanting genetically modified cells in the brain that produce nerve growth factor, a protein that prevents neuronal death and stimulates cell function. This gene therapy approach—which is being promoted by scientists at the University of California, San Diego, and the company they founded called Ceregene—enables scientists to create a designer stem cell. Rather than starting with stem cells, this treatment starts with skin cells called fibroblasts that are taken from individual patients. These cells are infected with a virus that has a copy of the nerve growth factor gene inserted into its genetic material, and then the cells are injected in a delicate operation near the cholinergic basal forebrain through a syringe.

The idea is that the fibroblasts, once introduced to the brain, will serve as tiny "pumps," producing nerve growth factor that has been shown to help mature neurons and mitigate degenerative cell death in cholinergic neurons and other cells important to thinking and learning. There is promise in this gene-therapy approach, but there are also reservations. The first are conceptual. With Alzheimer's, there is no one cell population in the brain that is singularly affected. Repairing cells in one or even several parts of the brain does not comprehensively treat the whole "disease" process.

Safety is also of concern. Perhaps the only condition that is worse than the uncontrolled *death* of brain cells is the uncontrolled *growth* of brain cells, as occurs in brain cancer. Introducing NGF into our brains could have the unintended consequence of causing tumors to form out of neural or other cells present in the brain, which possess NGF receptors. Researchers had attempted to add a tetracycline-responsive gene to the NGF virus that would serve as a switching-off mechanism and shut down production of NGF if it became excessive, but this technique has never worked well. Even beyond the risk of cancer, safety is an issue in the actual procedure itself, which requires neurosurgery in patients who are already prone to complications. Penetrating the brain with a needle can lead to fatal hemorrhaging, especially in older persons, who are more at risk for subdural hematoma, a blood clot on the brain. Two patients in human trials were said to have suffered brain damage when they moved during the procedure, and one died five weeks following the procedure.

AMYLOID VACCINE: THE OTHER GREAT HOPE

In addition to nerve cell replacement therapies like stem cells and NGF fibroblasts, most companies that study AD are focusing on dissolving beta-amyloid as the best hope, and contend that advances in genetic research will open up limitless possibilities for the development of new personalized drugs to treat AD. The amyloid cascade hypothesis has led to many approaches to prevent the formation, dissolve, or enhance clearance of amyloid. A rather surprising approach has focused on the production of amyloid antibodies to try to promote removal on the basis that the immune system naturally produces antibodies in response to damage. It was theorized that a vaccine could increase the body's production of amyloid antibodies, which may ultimately help prevent the widespread buildup of plaques. Dramatic results were found in transgenic mice models in which vaccines were used to reduce excessive amyloid. Transgenic animals are imperfect models of AD; nevertheless, those who pursue the amyloid hypothesis believe that they are still a good testing ground for medications.

A company called Elan, a large biotech firm with a long-standing, high-stakes investment in the neurological disease and the amyloid hypothesis, began drug trial testing rapidly after developing this therapeutic approach in their laboratory animals. Despite initial enthusiasm, the study was halted early when a significant percentage of participants in the trial developed an adverse reaction to the vaccine. The treatment had resulted in an allergic encephalitis, or inflammation of the brain, which led to the death of more than one patient and permanent damage in more.

THE DRUG DEVELOPMENT MACHINE LABORS ON

Despite the lack of results, Elan is spending a large amount of money to promote its efforts. For example, it hosted a large dinner for participants at the recent international Alzheimer's conference held in Madrid in July 2006. The hype associated with this approach continued to build, despite a lack of clear efficacy in the main analyses and permanent damage done to some patients.

Shortly after the trial was stopped, the company announced that the disappointing results would set their program back by less than a year. In fact, it took a considerably greater amount of time just to analyze the data. Only about 15 percent of participants actually developed an appropriate antibody response to the vaccine itself. In some of these subjects the vaccine appeared to contribute to some improvement in cognition over placebo. Those who appeared to respond to the vaccine with cognitive improvement had a greater degree of shrinkage of the brain on MRI scans. No one knows what caused this puzzling result. Perhaps because the amyloid was being cleared from the brain, the brain volume was reduced as a result. Whatever the case, this result was the opposite of what most people expected. The apparent clinical improvements were small and might have been due to chance, as in any study where there appears to be a subgroup of people who respond to a drug. We do not know if anyone in the study really benefited in a clinically meaningful way from the vaccine. The primary outcome measures for the study were in fact negative. In other words, some after-the-fact statistical analysis was required to claim that some people may have responded to the vaccine. These kinds of statistical approaches need to be viewed with caution, because they may find associations that are not replicated in other studies.

The dangers of active immunization, in which the patient is given the active amyloid antigen itself, have caused Elan and other companies to modify their active antigens and also develop trials of passive immunization. This therapy involves giving premade antibodies to individuals rather than having the individual's body produce them, as occurs with active immunization. Researchers at Cornell have tried administering intravenous immunoglobin (IVIG), which is a blood product obtained by pooling samples taken from many donors that contains the amyloid antibodies as well as a variety of other immunoglobulins. Initial, surprisingly positive results have been obtained in small numbers of patients, and larger trials of this approach are being planned. IVIG is exceedingly expensive, and widespread therapy using this approach is not likely to be a long-term solution.

ALZHEMED: THE AMYLOID DREDGING APPROACH

Alzhemed is an experimental oral product for mild-to-moderate AD that has been specifically designed to modify the course of the disease by binding to amyloid as the primary target, preventing the protein from forming into BAP deposits and filtering it out of the body.

Neurochem, which produces the drug, released results in 2004 showing that, overall, approximately 70 percent of the mild-AD patients had stabilized or improved cognitive function tests even after twenty months of enrollment in the Alzhemed open-label phase three extension study. The results were not so good for persons with moderate disease, as these patients continued to show signs of decline. Ultimately, the sample sizes of the study were too small to draw conclusions.

In drug trials, the process is divided into four stages. Phase one represents the first efforts to study drug metabolism; phase two is often the first introduction of patients with the illness to the drug; phase three represents larger studies undertaken for actual submission to regulatory bodies; phase four, or the "extension" period, is used to generate further safety data on the drug. The factors that make up a good study are: randomization of study participants into an intervention and control group, blind assessment (meaning that neither researcher nor participant knows who is in which group), well-defined outcomes and statistical plan, and careful entry criteria.

A fundamental critique of Alzhemed is that their treatment for Alzheimer's relies on the BAPtist belief that amyloid is the cause of AD. This may be an ill-defined target, since we aren't sure what role amyloid plays in brain aging. Since amyloid deposition may begin as early as the second or third decade, to be effective, Alzhemed might have to be given over the course of half of one's life! As it now stands, Alzhemed has not been administered long enough for us to track the long-term consequences of its action. The safety concerns for such a long administration are considerable.

As with all treatments, the short-term safety and tolerability of Alzhemed has also been brought into question. According to Neurochem, the company that makes the drug, Alzhemed appears to be safe and well tolerated after up to twenty months of follow-up, although the company reported that nausea and vomiting occurred at the beginning of the treatment and persisted in some cases for up to sixteen months. Overall, five patients withdrew prematurely from the beginning of the phase two clinical trial over the twenty-month period due to adverse events: three due to nausea and vomiting, one because of weakness and weight loss, and another for increased agitation and delusion. As I've mentioned before, it is always somewhat risky to disrupt the body's normal systems, especially with regard to a protein like amyloid precursor protein, which occurs throughout the body and may have neuroprotective properties. Alzhemed is still a long way from being a viable treatment. It has yet to receive FDA approval, and larger trials are now under way with the hope of putting the drug on the market in five years. Many in the field, including myself, are dubious of their ultimate success.

XALIPRODENE

Xaliprodene is a prospective neurotrophic treatment that has nerve growth factor (NGF)–like activity. Neurotrophins are small molecules that encourage the survival of nervous cells. Currently under development by Sanofi-Synthélabo, xaliprodene is being developed as an oral treatment for AD and Lou Gehrig's disease.

In cultures of glial cells, which provide support and nutrition to neurons, xaliprodene enhances the effects of NGF on cell survival and outgrowth and stimulates the production of NGF. Once again, the theoretical rationale appears reasonable, but the long-term benefits and safety remain to be determined. As with the cholinesterase inhibitors, we should be concerned about whether a therapy directed just at cholinergic, or more precisely nerve growth factor responsive, neurons will be effective enough to treat a multi-system disorder.

FLURIZAN

Flurizan (taurenflurbil) is being developed by Myriad Pharmaceuticals, a spin-off from the very profitable Myriad Genetics, which markets genetic and laboratory tests. The company believes that their compound binds to the gamma secretase and causes it to produce shorter forms of beta-amyloid. In other words, less of the 42-amino acid peptide is produced when the drug is active, sparing the brain from the supposedly toxic effects of the longer 42-amino acid protein. Evidence has been presented that the drug improves learning in mice whose brains have been modified to overproduce beta-amyloid by diminishing plaque accumulation. Preliminary clinical data in a small number of human beings is being interpreted by some as possibly slowing progression of disease. A phase three study with eight hundred subjects is under way to try to provide more definite evidence of effectiveness.

THE PHARMACEUTICAL INDUSTRY

In the past three decades, I've grown increasingly concerned by the disingenuous "overpromising" that goes on about treatments for Alzheimer's disease. Equally troubling is that the lofty rhetoric used by drug companies belies a profound failure of actual innovation toward new treatments. Despite the barrage of direct-to-consumer advertising you are exposed to that seems to suggest drug companies are producing a steady stream of innovative medicines, the success of the industry's research and development efforts has been slowing down just as genomics and a variety of other approaches have come along with the promise of improving the efficiency of drug development. Instead of being a highly beneficial-to-health industry that discovers and produces new treatments that may help assuage the hardships of brain aging, the industry has become too much of a marketing-driven entity that sells drugs of uncertain benefit at increasingly untenable prices and lobbies heavily for congressional favors.

Our pharmaceutical industry is in trouble, and its leadership knows it. At a meeting of the American College of Neuropsychopharmacology in Puerto Rico in December 2004, an executive of a major multinational told me that, quite frankly, "our business models are bankrupt and we will be, too, if we don't change them." Because drug companies have limited resources and perhaps limited intellectual and organizational flexibility for basic R&D, many of the advances in identifying new areas of research are actually occurring in the biotech industry and at universities. The pharmaceutical industry buys into this pioneering research by purchasing smaller companies. As Marcia Angell, a former editor in chief of *The New England Journal of Medicine* and a current member of Harvard Medical School's Department of Social Medicine, writes in her book *The Truth About the Drug Companies,* instead of being an engine of innovation for human health, the pharmaceutical industry is a "vast marketing machine" that is less of a free-market success story than one might think.[7] Like a freeloading, underachieving child still crashing at home, the industry lives off government-funded research and monopoly rights and is extravagantly rewarded for its less-than-stellar contributions. Most patients would probably be horrified if they knew how much money the pharmaceutical industry puts into providing meals, travel, parties, gift certificates, pens, and gadgets for doctors who prescribe their drugs. Consider this: The industry estimates that it spends approximately $5.7 billion on marketing to physicians. If you do the math, that means nearly six thousand dollars is being spent per doctor![8] This is money that could be applied to the development of drugs that could potentially help relieve the suffering of people all over the world. Big pharma is also one of the biggest spenders in Washington (and statehouses), hedging its bets by supporting both Republicans and Democrats. Add to their expense accounts all the lawyers they pay to defend intellectual property rights and to attack generic drugs, and it is a wonder that they have any money left to pay for actual research.

MY MESSAGE TO THE PHARMACEUTICAL INDUSTRY

Ten years ago I founded a group called the International Working Group for the Harmonization of Dementia Drug Guidelines. We succeeded in bringing together academics, industry leaders, and government regulators to discuss Alzheimer's and related disorders and helped craft guidelines necessary to demonstrate that a drug should be approved for the treatment of Alzheimer's disease. Not only did we focus on drugs, we also explored pharmaco-economic issues, considered ethical and cultural issues that affected drug development, and brought attention to the need to improve the efficiency of drug development around the world.

The governing bodies that oversee the health of our citizens must challenge the pharmaceutical industry to spur real innovation and turn out products that lengthen life, enhance its quality, and sustain cognitive vitality.

Further, it is time for society to apply pressure on the pharmaceutical industry and the medical profession so dominated by it, and press them to change their way of doing business. Professional medical societies should lead their members back on a more ethically palatable path, but even their own budgets are often quite dependent on industry funding—that's how enmeshed medicine is in big pharma.

Major responsibility falls on the shoulders of our national and international regulatory bodies: They have the task of setting the standards required for drug approval and monitoring the behavior of the pharmaceutical industry. Regulators must limit the priority given to minimally effective drugs such as cholinesterase inhibitors, and priority should be given to new chemical entities. The pharmaceutical industry can play a vital role in the future of brain aging, but it must accept its mantle of responsibility and work as an agent of world benefit. While a biological cure for Alzheimer's disease may be beyond our human capability, we must harness the power of the drug industry to seek genuinely effective treatments that will improve our quality of life as we age.

THE NEED FOR A DEEP BIOETHICS

The relationship between the medical profession and the health industry (device manufacturers and drug companies) is problematic to say the least. Arthur Kleinman, the famous medical anthropologist from Harvard, has called the corrupted partnership the greatest ethical problem in medicine today. Personally, I find the lapses in ethical behavior in the medical profession distressing. After all, we expect businesses to try to sell their products, and improve their bottom line. Conversely, we expect medical professionals to fulfill their social contract and to give counsel about health—not to help sell pills and devices. Redressing the problematic relationship between medicine and industry and establishing an ethical synergy is one of the greatest issues facing modern medicine—an issue that I wish the newly emergent field of bioethics was more proactive in tackling.

Bioethics is a nascent field that is only twenty-five years old. One of my mentors in bioethics, V. R. Potter, was the first to coin the term.[9] Potter identified the need for an interdisciplinary effort to understand the role and responsibilities of the human species for the planet, and to head off ethical transgressions that might be engendered by the profit motive in medicine. I started my career as a professor of bioethics studying and writing on such issues as genetic testing, informed consent in patients with cognitive impairment, and end-of-life care. I became so interested that I went on to earn a master's degree from my current university. However, I soon grew disenchanted by bioethics when I began to see how co-opted it had become by the medical profession, and how uncritical it was of the malfeasance and questionable conduct of current medical practice. Bioethicists can be legitimate watchdogs for the public, but they must commit themselves to tackling the salient issues that are affecting the practice of medicine and corroding our health-care system.

THE POWER OF STORIES

There's an old story told about three blind men who came upon an elephant in India. Not knowing what the creature was, each man laid his hands upon a different part of its body. One man stroked the elephant's side and exclaimed, "Well, well, this beast is exactly like a wall." The second felt only the elephant's tusk and said, "My friend, you are mistaken, it feels more like a spear than a wall." The third happened to take hold of the elephant's tail and declaimed, "You are both wrong. Anyone with an ounce of sense could see that this creature is like a snake."

The moral of course is that humans often fail to observe objects in their holistic complexity. When this story is seen as an allegory of modern genetic medicine, we are reminded that Western medical practice is often guilty of the myopia of the men in the story. Genetic reductionism has not led us to the promised land of personalized medicine. By ignoring the totality of the human experience—the moral, psychosocial, ethical, cultural, spiritual dimensions of life and the environmental and lifestyle factors that contribute to health and disease—and attempting to reduce us to our genes, or to a single therapeutic target (amyloid, the cholinergic forebrain, and so on), Western medicine is failing to address the complexities of human beings living in communities. Alzheimer's disease cannot be reduced to a purely molecular substrate—the story of brain aging is not so simple.

In Cleveland, we are launching a project called StoryBank to collect patient stories and other health narratives in parallel with a biobank that intends to store DNA and extracted tissues donated by persons in northeast Ohio. As I mentioned, at Johns Hopkins I created and managed the Brain Resource Center, a type of biobank (for brains) to support our work on cholinergic and other systems in Alzheimer's disease, and so I know the power of an interdisciplinary neuroscientific approach to analyzing cells and genes in tissues collected at autopsy. This enterprise helped make my career by allowing me to collaborate with many other investigators interested in studying our donated tissues. I see a similar synergy with StoryBank.

While genetic biomedicine clearly offers some hope for helping human beings cope with health challenges, our greatest hope is to be found in our interconnectedness as humans. We can't promise our dementia patients that we will be able to "fix" their brains with stem cells or other miracle interventions; but we can honor them in the midst of their suffering by truly engaging and bearing witness to their story and gaining wisdom from it. A focus on individual narratives can bring personal stories from people's lives into prominence over the standard, reductionist, totalizing myths of conditions like Alzheimer's disease. It can also begin to uncover the manifold environmental and lifestyle inputs of brain aging that affect people throughout our lives, and suggest how we might be better able to shape a public-health message about prevention.

Indeed, StoryBank is not merely an academic project, it represents an attempt to improve public health in Cleveland and beyond. Such a focus on personal and community narrative is sorely needed to countervail against the reductionism of biomedicine. Indeed, unlike the three blind men, healers of aging patients in the twenty-first century must begin to widen their ken to perceive the "elephant in the room" in its full complexity rather than narrowing their gaze merely on degenerating brains, or on the genes that encode for proteins that gather on those brains. The paradigm of care must shift toward "wholism." We must begin to see persons with aging brains through a holistic, ecological lens—StoryBank promises to do so.

We must remember that molecular genetics is but one small part of the story of cognitive change, and that brain aging is but one small part of what makes us human. Despite the "mythical" misinformation so prevalent in our media about genetic risk and up-and-coming molecular cures, there is no simple breakthrough cure that will "fix" our aging brains—not even on the horizon. This should not be grounds for consternation. In some ways, the lack of genetic determinism should inspire hope in us, for there is much that we can do to promote our cognitive wellness as we age.

PART THREE

A New Model for Living with Brain Aging

CHAPTER SEVEN

IDENTIFYING WHO NEEDS A PRESCRIPTION FOR MEMORY LOSS

Blessed are the forgetful: for they get the better even of their blunders.

—FRIEDRICH NIETZSCHE

Many years ago, I stood staring at my door, Room 212, in the palatial Prince Hotel in Osaka, Japan, with a look of confusion on my face. I'd flown into Japan in the morning for an international conference on Alzheimer's disease and had been racked by jet lag the whole day. That night I wanted to get a little rest. The only thing preventing me from entering my room was a malfunctioning electronic key that kept refusing me entrance. I slipped the key in and out of the reader. I jiggled the door handle. I nudged my shoulder into the door. It was all to no avail. The room remained locked.

Weary, exhausted, and grumpy from a day of travel, I marched down to the lobby and set the key on the front desk.

"It doesn't work," I said to the attendant with exasperation.

He looked down at my card and then up at me.

"What room are you in, sir?" he asked in heavily accented English, to which I replied, "Two-twelve."

He smiled, read my name off my name tag, and typed it into his computer.

"Dr. Whitehouse has Room *Three*-twelve," he said.

Realizing my mistake, I laughed to myself, bowed sheepishly, and went back upstairs to find my real bed.

We all have "senior moments" like this.

Who among us hasn't experienced an inexplicable memory lapse that has aroused anxiety about Alzheimer's disease? In Japan they call transient states of confusion like my hotel room mishap by a specific name: *boke*. Moments of *boke* provoke anxiety among the Japanese, but because they are often attributed to the vagaries of normal aging, they are not entirely unexpected and are not spoken of in the same breath as dementia. At times, the condition is evoked as a source of humor by comedians and on television shows; generally, affected persons are depicted in the public media in a cute way, much like a dependent child.[1]

As we grow older, we can expect more moments of *boke* in our lives as well. Whether that means occasionally forgetting dates, misplacing keys and cell phones, losing words and names on the tip of your tongue, or storming around outside someone else's hotel door in Osaka like a modern-day Godzilla, we can expect that these events will become more common as our bodies and minds age.

Although occasional memory slippage may be a normal consequence of getting older, when memory problems begin to interfere with your day-to-day activities there is a fine line between casually dismissing slippages and needing to seek a doctor's help. One of the more distressing dilemmas we all face as we age is whether to seek medical care for our brain aging. Although there is no clear-cut line between normal changes and warning signs, there are commonsense approaches to determine whether you or a loved one should visit a doctor.

ASSESSING MEMORY CHALLENGES IN YOUR FAMILY

In the early 1990s I was part of a team of clinicians who developed a ten-point checklist for the Alzheimer's Association of common symptoms to help people recognize the difference between normal age-related memory changes and possible warning signs for dementia. When we were developing it, I was a bit concerned because it was produced with a grant from the company that made tacrine, the first drug approved for the treatment of Alzheimer's disease. I wondered in fact whether we were really putting together the ten warning signs that would qualify you as a tacrine customer! Nearly two decades later, I have updated and clarified this checklist to enable you to decide whether you need to seek professional help for your memory loss or encourage some someone else to.

Ten warning signs of cognitive impairment requiring medical attention:[2]

> Memory loss
> Difficulty performing familiar tasks
> Problems with language
> Disorientation to time and place
> Poor or decreased judgment
> Problems with abstract thinking
> Misplacing things
> Changes in mood or behavior
> Changes in personality
> Loss of initiative

Memory loss

The Alzheimer's Association considers forgetting recently learned information one of the most common early signs of dementia, which is true to an extent. Though it's normal for people of all ages to forget appointments, names, or telephone numbers on occasion, those with problematic brain aging will forget such information more often and cannot recall it later, even with the help of cues.

What's normal? It is practically impossible to define what is normal, because everyone brings different cognitive abilities into their old age. A good rule of thumb is to measure the loss in function against the level of function you or a loved one had when you were younger. If you are losing words on the tip of your tongue but were not that great of a speaker in the first place, your situation may not be so dire. If words always came easily to you but now sentences are a struggle, your problem may require medical attention. Generally speaking, we are not very good judges of our own cognitive decline. It is often helpful to have someone who knows us well give us their opinion of whether they feel our memory loss is normal or not. Such opinions should be ventured in a manner that is frank, but uncritical.

> *The advantage of a bad memory is that one enjoys several times the same good things for the first time.*
> —FRIEDRICH NIETZSCHE

Difficulty performing familiar tasks

According to the Alzheimer's Association, people with dementia often find it hard to plan or complete everyday tasks. This is a telltale sign of cognitive decline. Individuals may lose track of the steps involved in preparing a meal, placing a telephone call, operating a household appliance, or participating in a game or lifetime hobby—activities that fall under the procedural memory category. We all will occasionally go into the basement and forget what we went down for. A person with dementia may forget at times that the basement is their own (autobiographical or episodic memory) and become disoriented to both time and place.

What's normal? Again, what is normal is a matter of degree. Occasionally forgetting why you came into a room or what you planned to say is something that happens to us all. The key questions to ask are:

- With what frequency are these mishaps occurring?
- Are they troubling or endangering you or those around you?
- Is your inability to perform the tasks of everyday life impinging on your quality of life, or that of your loved ones?

It is often the case that memory problems affect caregivers more than the patients themselves. For instance, many of my patients perseverate (repeat themselves). Though they are unaware of their repetition, it is often extremely wearing on their caregivers. Consequently, caregivers are often the best judges of normalcy, and it is wise to defer to their expertise.

Problems with language

People with dementia often forget simple words or substitute unusual words called "neologisms," making their speech or writing difficult to understand. The Alzheimer's Association gives the example of a person unable to find her toothbrush who instead asks for "that thing for my mouth" or uses garbled phrases to request it. With my patients, the most common problem is not making up new words but forgetting old ones. This process of word-finding difficulty creates pauses in conversation, and can result in patients using circumlocutions to try to get around the memory gap.

What's normal? Whether we are in the bloom of youth or great-grandparents, we all sometimes have trouble finding the right words. If you or a loved one can't come up with the word for toothbrush, this problem is far more benign than if unusual words or neologisms are substituted in its place. Again, our language malfunction should be interpreted relative to our functioning in the past. The decline of our cognitive functioning is inevitable; the *steepness* of the decline is what matters.

Disorientation to time and place

People with dementia can become lost in their own neighborhood, lose comprehension of where they are and how they got there, and be incapable of getting themselves back home. Quite often, my patients and their care-givers will tell me that such an incident was what finally compelled them to seek medical attention. Unfortunately, it usually involves getting lost in a car. I remember one of my patients who came to see me after making a wrong turn on an expressway and ending up in Buffalo, New York, rather than Cleveland. That's quite a mistake, the magnitude of which well warrants medical attention.

What's normal? As the Alzheimer's Association suggests, forgetting the day of the week or where you were going is an understandable lapse of orientation in a busy and chaotic modern world. We must ask questions about the magnitude of the disorientation.

- Are you getting lost on the Tokyo subway system or in your own home?

- And under what circumstances did you get lost?

- Have you not been getting enough sleep?

- Was alcohol, stress, depression, or medication involved?

- How often is it happening? Now and then? Once a week?

The answers to such questions can help you sort out whether a trip to the doctor is needed. If you notice that a loved one is increasingly incapable of navigating through his life—especially if his confusion is endangering him and others—some "tough love" may be needed. It is difficult to question another's ability to function in the world, but the costs of intervening are far outweighed by the benefits. Frankness and empathy are the best tools to use in such situations.

THE IMPORTANCE OF SLEEP

It is believed that memories are consolidated by the brain during rapid eye movement (REM) sleep. Thus, sleep deprivation can cause difficulties in the storage and recall process, which is why you may not feel quite as sharp after a night of tossing and turning. Though everyone varies in their sleeping patterns, a good rule of thumb for keeping your memory strong day to day is to make sure you keep regular sleeping habits and get seven or so hours a night. The International Longevity Center-USA, a research policy organization in New York City led by my friend and colleague Bob Butler, recently released its sleep and healthy aging tips for older adults, which offer comprehensive advice:

Do:

- Go to bed at the same time each night, and get up and out of bed at the same time each morning.

- Keep your bedroom/sleeping area dark, cool, quiet, restful, and comfortable.

- If you cannot fall asleep within twenty minutes, get out of bed and read something boring until you feel sleepy.

- Engage in physical activity, outdoors if possible, during the day (at least four hours before bedtime).

- Take a hot bath sixty to ninety minutes before bedtime.

- Listen to soft or soothing music.

- Use visualization—picture a relaxing scene.

Do not:

- Drink caffeinated beverages for at least six hours before going to bed (this includes coffee, tea, and soda).
- Drink alcohol at bedtime or for two hours before bedtime; daytime alcohol consumption should be in moderation.
- Smoke cigarettes at least four hours before bedtime (of course, it's best not to smoke at all).
- Fall asleep with the television on.
- Exercise within four hours of going to bed.
- Read stimulating material while in bed just before turning out the lights.
- Take a long nap during the day (more than thirty minutes).
- Go to bed too hungry or too full. If you are hungry, a light carbohydrate snack (e.g., crackers with milk) may help.

To read the whole report see: www.ilcuse.org/lib/pdf/sleep&healthy aging.pdf.

Poor or decreased judgment

Those with dementia may dress inappropriately, or show poor judgment in various aspects of their lives that doesn't fit with previous behavior. A common warning sign that we see in our clinic is patients who give away large sums of money to telemarketers or pay for home repairs or superfluous products they don't need. I remember a patient who came to see me a few years ago because he was obsessing about his mail. He would compulsively respond to sweepstakes mailings, and, after several months, had become listed on countless mailing distribution lists. As a result, more and more of these sweepstakes scams trickled in through the mail, giving him more and more opportunities to squander his money—something he would have never done had he been of sound judgment.

What's normal? Making a questionable or debatable decision about personal finance from time to time is something we are all guilty of.

- Are your mistakes egregious enough that other people begin to take notice?

- Are you able to understand and express your lapse in reasoning and learn from it?

Those who are unaware of their reasoning errors may have more serious problems and may need others to intervene in their affairs and help them seek medical attention. Again, it is necessary to measure a person's mishaps against her past behavior. Has she always been prone to bad judgment? Or has she always been sharp as a tack? Family and friends are in the best position to make such judgment calls.

Problems with abstract thinking

Someone with dementia, the Alzheimer's Association suggests, may have unusual difficulty performing complex mental tasks such as remembering what numbers are for and how they should be used. In my experience, the main problem linked with this particular cognitive challenge often involves lapses in maintaining family banking accounts.

What's normal? We might say that it's normal to find such an activity as balancing a checkbook a challenge. This is not an easy task for anyone, and complications do not necessarily signal a cognitive problem requiring medical attention. If you or a loved one simply lacks the ability to engage with numbers, and if this confusion is sustained and creates mounting frustration, it is important that you seek medical attention. There may be cognitive factors other than dementia that are impinging on your cognitive functioning. A doctor can help determine if any of these factors are confounding your ability to think abstractly.

Misplacing things

A person with Alzheimer's disease may put things in unusual places. For instance, Dr. Alzheimer noted that at the start of Auguste D.'s decline she began storing her mail in boxes beneath her bed. The patients I care for who have dementia often lose their glasses, their purses, or other everyday items with consistency. Some become obsessive collectors of bric-a-brac, and will store objects in peculiar places. For instance, I remember a patient that I cared for in-home who had accumulated so many newspapers in her apartment that it became a fire and health hazard.

What's normal? Misplacing keys, a wallet, or a purse temporarily is something that happens to everyone, regardless of age (having raised three daughters, I can say this with authority!). It is essential to ask with what frequency objects are being misplaced. If it happens a couple times a week, it may not be so serious, but if objects—especially the same objects—are being mislaid with consistency, the problem may be more urgent. You must consider whether a loved one is using the appropriate problem-solving strategies to backtrack and figure out where an object was mislaid. A clear ability to recapitulate your past actions shows a strong and stable memory that may not necessitate medical help.

A key determining factor for seeking medical care hinges on whether the person tends to blame others for their misplaced possessions or whether they accept responsibility. Making baseless accusations, as Auguste D. did in accusing her husband of going on walks with another woman, can be a sign of frontal lobe dementia. Accepting blame and reflecting on reasons for a mishap is a sign of cognitive health. Caching newspapers in bizarre places around the house is a sign that there may be an underlying condition that requires medical consultation.

Changes in mood or behavior

Everyone can become sad or moody from time to time. Someone with dementia may show rapid mood swings—from calm to tears to anger—for no apparent reason. Indeed, from Chapter 3 recall that Dr. Alzheimer described Auguste D. as becoming lachrymose and tearful without the slightest bit of provocation. Indeed, common symptoms that we see in the elderly are abrupt bouts of depression, psychosis, irritability, wandering, agitation, and aggression. In particular, depression coexists with Alzheimer's. After all, learning to adjust to a cognitive impairment would be an emotional challenge for us all. The most hard-to-read patients are those who have had a tendency toward depression for much of their life. Sorting out how much dementia is due to depression and how much is due to cognitive aging is often a challenge. In my experience, families are usually the best judges of this since they can use a loved one's past as a reference point for assessing current decline.

What's normal? We all occasionally feel melancholy and antisocial. But if a person shows uncharacteristically morose behavior over a sustained period of time, or if they show catastrophic reactions that are out of character and disproportionate to the stimulus, these are usually signs that there are more serious cognitive challenges requiring medical attention. We must measure our assessment against past behavior. Was your father a calm and even-keeled person but is now flying off the handle at the slightest perturbation? Or conversely, was your mom an irascible and aggressive woman in her youth but is now sad and sedate? Behavioral changes point to a frontal lobe dementia or could be symptoms of depression, which can be treated medically. Again, the steepness of the slope is what is important to gauge rather than the slope itself.

CREATING A NEW DISEASE SYNDROME

For many decades neurologists have been aware of a condition called pseudobulbar affect (PBA). This syndrome refers to the sudden outburst of crying or laughing that occurs involuntarily and without strong underlying subjective emotion in conditions like multiple sclerosis and amyotrophic lateral sclerosis. A pharmaceutical company called Avanir is developing a physician education campaign focusing on broadening conceptions of PBA to potentially expand the market to patients with dementia. The company is supporting efforts to develop a new term, "Involuntary Emotional Expression Disorder (IEED)," that would include PBA and perhaps other more general categories such as emotional incontinence and emotional lability. Such a classification would create potentially millions more consumers for their drug, which has not yet been approved by the FDA. A *New York Times* article even suggested that people with road rage should consider this medication! If the drug helps at a reasonable cost, it would be great. However, the first line of management of PBA is to make people aware that these involuntary emotional outbursts are well-described phenomena and are not associated with an underlying depression.

Changes in personality

As many of us know, the day-to-day behaviors of persons with dementia can be quite variable. But do their basic personalities change? While people do not "lose themselves," they may come to display character traits or features that strike us as unusual and uncharacteristic. Some common behaviors I often observe in my patients are suspicion, anxiety, and obsessiveness. In dementia, people's negative features tend to be amplified rather than their more likable features, although the caregivers of my patients often tell me that they are enjoying the new mellowed-out version of their parent. In fact, some children of persons with dementia are grateful for the opportunity to rebuild a strained relationship with a parent on different terms.

What's normal? People's personalities can change with age, but, again, more drastic changes require that we act with greater urgency. Some warning signs to look for are whether someone is markedly less flexible, less novelty-seeking, or far more sluggish than he used to be. Similarly, if a person was always a bit restrained and is now growing more agitated and aggressive, this is a red flag for caregivers to act on. Physical violence is a major red flag. Although we tend to approach changes in character from a "medicalized" perspective, it is equally important to remember that we change at every stage of our lives. Certainly, many of us look back with incredulity at the behaviors, values, and worldviews we embodied in our teens or early twenties. On the other hand, getting older can open up freedom in behavior not present early in life. As Shakespeare wrote in *As You Like It,* old age is a sort of "second childishness . . . sans teeth, sans eyes, sans taste, sans everything."

> *People think it's a terrible tragedy when somebody has Alzheimer's. But in my mother's case, it's different. My mother has been unhappy all her life. . . . For the first time in her life, she's happy.*
>
> —AMY TAN

Loss of initiative

It's normal to tire mentally of housework, business activities, or social obligations at times. A person with troublesome brain aging may become very passive, sitting in front of the TV for long stretches of time, sleeping more than usual, or not wanting to do activities that they've long enjoyed. One of the hardest things to judge is the amount of activity that is appropriate. Caregivers often have a hard time adjusting to the fact that somebody with dementia may need and want to lead a simpler life.

What's normal? Feeling weary of work or social obligations on occasion is normal, if not expected. A key question to ask is whether the patient has insight into their own problem or whether a caregiver must make this determination on their behalf. Those who lack the capacity to reflect inwardly on the reasons for their loss of initiative should be encouraged to receive medical care. A loss of initiative may be due to medical illnesses, including simple things like dehydration, or cardiovascular problems that people can easily miss, which are easily treatable.

WHEN YOU SEE WARNING SIGNS

If you recognize any warning signs in yourself or a loved one, the Alzheimer's Association recommends consulting a doctor. In my opinion, before doing that, it's wise to talk to others to see if they are concerned. If people close to you feel that a decline is apparent, a consultation with a doctor should be a strong consideration. The main thing to look for is a marked change from a prior state that is unrecognized by the affected person. The decline is of more concern if it is affecting activities of daily living, or if safety is a recurring issue.

From a practical standpoint, you or someone close to you should keep a diary that lists your range and progression of symptoms, highlighting the worst that has happened over the course of your decline. It helps a physician to have a chronological understanding of when events have happened to you, and to ascertain specific details about their frequency and magnitude.

Before you talk to a medical specialist—neurologist, geriatrician, or psychiatrist—I recommend that you address your concerns with a primary-care physician and discuss how your memory problems are affecting your health. But if your physician is uncomfortable discussing these issues or doesn't fulfill your need for information, then the proper thing to do would be to ask for a referral to a specialist. There may be other underlying physiological causes that manifest as the symptoms of brain aging, including: hypothyroidism, vascular disease, vitamin and micronutrient deficiencies, depression, fatigue, grief, dehydration, vision or hearing loss, alcohol use, complications from diabetes, from epilepsy, and from medications, or chronic stress. These alternative causes—which clinicians call "differential diagnoses"—can often be treated by your physician, and may reverse apparent symptoms of brain aging before you need to go through the trouble of making an appointment to see a specialist.

CONSIDERING THE DIFFERENTIAL DIAGNOSES OF BRAIN AGING

Depression. This condition slows down brain function and can make it difficult to process new memories other than those involving fear and sadness. It has also been claimed to lead to frontal lobe dysfunction, shrinkage of the hippocampus, and/or damage to nerve structure at the subcortical level,[3] and has been associated with increased numbers of plaques and tangles[4] and more rapid cognitive decline. Fortunately, depression can be treated bio-psychosocially, with medications and therapy.

Hypothyroidism. Because the thyroid gland regulates virtually every metabolic process in the body, an alteration in its output can have major effects on human functioning. Additionally, some studies suggest thyroid activity affects both the structure of the hippocampus and the enzymes present in the brain that regulate the metabolic rate of neurons, so impaired functioning can lead to mental lethargy, memory loss, depression, anxiety, and fatigue. Once hypothyroidism is detected, doctors can readily treat it with a hormone replacement therapy.

Epilepsy. If you or a loved one is epileptic and taking anticonvulsant drugs, these medications can slow the brain down and cause memory problems. Doctors can usually address this problem by checking levels of the drug in the blood and finding the right dosage for patients or changing the medication. In rare cases, seizures themselves can cause intermittent memory problems.

Calcium deficiency (hypocalcaemia). Calcium helps maintain neuronal membrane excitability, meaning that it enables fast and efficient transmission of signals between neurons. In this way, it helps regulate neuronal metabolism and neurotransmitter synthesis and release. A shortage of calcium can bring about neuronal malfunction. If diagnosed, it is readily treated by identifying the cause and providing supplementation.

Alcoholism. The brains of alcoholics show structural changes as well as physiological impairment (reduced cerebral blood flow and altered electrical brain waves). These changes can also be linked to nutritional deficits because people who are drinking heavily obtain most of their calories from nutrition-depleted beer and liquor. There is evidence that if people stop drinking and commit to a rehabilitation program, they can recover from some if not all of the impairment caused by their drinking. But until a person stops drinking, their long- and short-term memories can be adversely affected by alcohol consumption.

WHAT YOU SHOULD YOU DO IF YOUR LOVED ONE RESISTS YOUR SUGGESTION TO SEEK MEDICAL HELP FOR MEMORY LOSS

This problem weighs on many caregivers. If an agreement can't be reached, a small amount of deception may be required. The most common strategy I recommend is to encourage your loved one to seek a general medical checkup with his primary-care physician but de-emphasize the memory problems. Meanwhile, call ahead to the physician and alert her to your loved one's memory problems so that the doctor can make preparations for a screening during the visit.

KNOWING THE TERRITORY OF THE BRAIN

Getting familiar with and accepting of the symptoms of brain aging is far more important in our lives than comprehending the underlying physiology of brain aging, but it may be helpful to know a little bit more about how and why the brain ages.

The brain begins to show signs of aging quite early in life. The facility for learning new languages actually tapers off sometime before adolescence, and we begin to accumulate plaques and tangles on our brains as early as our twenties or thirties. As we enter early adulthood, brain atrophy begins to occur due to the loss of neurons and hormonal changes (including those engendered by stress) that affect brain chemistry and blood flow to our brains. In midlife there is an observable decline in everyone's raw mental agility—the ability to recall lists of objects, group objects into classes, and replace words with numbers (or vice versa).

The speed of reaction to the world is also compromised. As the brain grows older in our latter decades, it undergoes complex biochemical, molecular, structural, and functional changes that are poorly understood by modern science. After we hit fifty, our brains further decrease in volume and weight by about 5 percent each decade, and this shrinkage and neuronal loss, although universal, affects people's mental performance in different ways.[5] Sensory organs feeding information to the brain also change with age. As we all know from our own lives, we gradually lose our ability to:

- Hear higher frequencies

- See—our eyesight becomes less sensitive and acute

- Detect a range of smells

- Form new memories

- Learn motor skills and react quickly

- Thermo-regulate (maintain our body's temperature)

"OH, YOU MUST BE . . ."

After age thirty, we tend to show a steady decrease in our ability to recall names. Here are a few tips to help you remember the names of people you meet:

1. Pay attention: Don't be distracted by other people or thoughts.

2. Repeat the name back to the person: Repetition helps solidify the name and face in your neuronal network.

3. Reference the person's name to an image, song lyric, etc.: Creating an association to an existing memory will increase the likelihood of you storing the new information.

> 4. Link the person's name to the name of a person you already know: If you meet a man named George, link him with George Bush, George Harrison, or Daniel George, the co-author of *The Myth of Alzheimer's*!
>
> 5. After you've met the person, take a few seconds and try to digest the essential information about him: This is called creating a schema, or mental framework, in which to fit the new information.

Thus, as we age we ask people to repeat themselves in conversations. We wear reading glasses to compensate for our failing vision and have trouble driving at night. We can't hit a tennis ball or catch our son's fastball like we once did. We layer up in the winter and may crank the air-conditioning up in the summer. We use cheat sheets and mnemonics, PDAs and other electronic devices to help hold memories and information that our minds can't cling to.

Some people are unaffected on the surface by these molecular changes. Everyone has a "sharp as a tack" relative who seems inoculated against the ravages of aging. Others struggle daily to remember where they put the house keys or parked the car. No single mechanism adequately explains why some brains age differently than others. And even those that are "sharp as a tack" probably do not think as quickly, but they compensate by using experience and well-routinized cognitive strategies.

As you know from "Alzheimer's 101," some scientists talk about the oxidative stress caused by free radicals and some propose inflammatory processes to explain neural senescence. Still others suggest that brain aging could be caused by changes in the way genes are expressed, the failure to properly remove beta-amyloid proteins, a decrease in neurotransmitters such as acetylcholine, dopamine, and serotonin, and dysfunction among the neurons' mitochondria, the small components in our cells that provide them with energy.[6] All the mechanisms used to explain normal brain aging have also been implicated as causes for Alzheimer's disease, suggesting that there is no separate disease process to differentiate AD from brain aging.

A REASON TO BE OPTIMISTIC ABOUT AGING

Despite the universal process of brain aging, we are finding that the aging brain is still quite possibly capable of growing some types of new cells and certainly of making connections between them, especially in the hippocampus. Recent studies on rats show that new neuronal cells are generated in older brains, but that these cells are retained only by rats that engage in active learning to build synaptic connections between the cells.[7] Subsequent studies have produced evidence that increased environmental complexity stimulates the growth of new hippocampal neurons (i.e., neurogenesis) in the adult brains of various species, such as birds, rodents, primates, and humans. Thus, neuroscience's long-held belief that there can be no addition of neurons in the adult mammalian brain has recently been revised.[8]

The lesson from these studies reinforces the old "Use it or lose it" axiom. More important, the studies demonstrate that our brain plasticity—the ability to continually generate cells and adapt to new and changing circumstances—enables us to engage in lifelong learning and stay cognitively vital as we grow older. I should add that the phrase "use it or lose it" is more of an optimistic hope than an empirical reality proven by science. While there is no firm evidence that engaging in mentally challenging activities can improve your brain directly, it still makes sense to live your life in an active and vital way.

SIZE DOESN'T MATTER

Many years ago, a neurologist colleague at Johns Hopkins, who had done his residency at Harvard, shared with me his story of brain shrinkage. At Harvard, he participated in a neuroimaging protocol as a volunteer. A scan was taken of his brain that showed moderate atrophy of brain tissue, which filled him with great anxiety. However, he remained exceptionally intelligent, and went on to a highly successful career. The lesson in this story is that it is not so important what our brains look like as they age. It's what we do with them that counts.

What if you don't recognize any symptoms of brain aging, but are still concerned about your memory? One solution is to request a memory screening from your physician. This is a simple, noninvasive procedure that can help give you a clear picture of your memory challenges and might allay your anxiety altogether. When I perform basic memory screenings with my patients I simply ask them to remember three words (such as *red, magazine,* and *Chevrolet*) for a minute or so and then give them graded clues if they cannot remember these words immediately. For example, I first give semantic clues. Was it a color? Was it a type of car? And then I try multiple choice. Was it the color red, blue, or green? It is a quick but sensitive way to get a read on the extent of a person's memory loss. If you want, you could ask a friend or family member to administer such a challenge to you, or you could take a test on a Web site. However, judgment is required in interpreting the results of any test (some test takers get very anxious when challenged in this direct way). I certainly wouldn't recommend self-diagnosis, and am skeptical of online diagnostic tests.

Emerging elders—including myself—are all going to suffer from bouts of cognitive impairment and perhaps even chronic loss as we age. Our condition does not require immediate medical attention but our memory challenges may eventually grow serious enough for us to seek medical consultation from a physician.

CHAPTER EIGHT

PREPARING FOR A DOCTOR'S VISIT

To write prescriptions is easy, but to come to an understanding with people is hard.

—FRANZ KAFKA

A few years ago, one of my colleagues became concerned about my hyperactivity. I've always been an energetic guy, and often joke about living more than one life in parallel. My colleague was so flabbergasted by my energy level that he approached the chief of staff at our hospital and recommended that I receive a medical evaluation.

Under intense confidentiality, I was asked to make an appointment with a psychiatrist. Although I was not concerned myself, since my father, a pediatrician, and other family members have a tendency toward hyperactivity, I decided to go forward with the procedure and use it as a learning opportunity.

Before my visit, I began to feel some pangs of concern. What if I got labeled with some disease? What if I was called hypomanic or even manic? Fortunately, the psychiatrist turned out to be an understanding man who took the time to sit down and talk with me and assess the situation. Our discussion served to calm my concerns. Instead of labeling me with a medical illness, he helped me to celebrate my active, effervescent nature and reminded me that there were many people in the academic world with high energy levels.

Inevitably, as we age, we will all have to confront the medical establishment at some time or another. Our brains are the most fragile organs in our bodies, and as they get older, the changes mentioned throughout the book occur in almost everyone to one degree or another. Your memory becomes less sharp. Your sleeping habits change. Your vision and hearing aren't what they used to be. Words and names don't come as easily or quickly.

When these changes begin to occur, it is natural to want to seek out medical care for your brain aging, and even more natural to fear as I did what you might find out when you visit the doctor. However, our anxieties about seeing a doctor are often unfounded.

Clinicians address health-related concerns and welcome the opportunity to guide patients and families through the changing circumstances we all must face sometime or another. Truly skilled clinicians will make you feel comfortable and will listen to what you need to express and help you adapt to your condition rather than focusing only on diagnosis and medical treatment.

Having determined to seek medical care, you now have to find a doctor who will assist you in developing the story by which you and your loved ones will live your later years. Once you find your doctor, how do you make sure that you and your family are organized and prepared for your visit, and that you ask the right kind of questions before, during, and after your appointment?

FINDING THE RIGHT HEALTH TEAM

Whether you are seeking care for yourself or for a loved one, the search for a good doctor is not always easy. The key is to maintain your composure and common sense, use the resources at your disposal, and realize that you are not alone and that you are in control of the situation. You have friends and family to help you through this process, and there are nonprofit organizations committed to assisting you in finding the right health team.

Practically speaking, your first step ought to be to check your insurance to find out whom they'll pay for you to visit. Even if your insurance won't pay for a doctor you wish to see or requires a co-pay, it is still worth considering a visit if the clinician comes highly recommended. Sometimes people decide to see me without clearance from their insurance company. I have few qualms about waiving my professional fees for the initial assessment, if the circumstances warrant it (which is appreciated by those financially challenged patients but not by my financially challenged employers), but this is not to be expected from every doctor.

Next, you should ask your primary-care physician to provide advice about your memory challenge or other cognitive symptoms. Some patients come to see me because they felt they could not adequately talk about their memory problems with their regular physician; others seek me out because they felt their concerns were not taken seriously enough, or because they were concerned that their physician lacked experience in dealing with aging issues. If you come to the conclusion that your physician is not treating your situation with sufficient skill, openness, or gravity, you should seek out the advice of anyone close to you who has dealt with similar issues before. Many of my referrals come from word-of-mouth recommendations, from people who have either come to see me or heard about my practice through the grapevine.

This grassroots approach to finding a physician has many benefits. My patients are more comfortable coming to see a highly recommended doctor, which helps to establish an initial trust even before the patient and I see each other. If, however, you are not familiar with anyone who has sought out medical care for memory problems, there are several important organizations committed to helping you locate highly regarded clinicians. The one to whom most people turn is the Alzheimer's Association (AA). Though I quibble with the name and aims of the organization, the local chapters of the AA usually do a good job providing core services to families, including information and referral, support groups, care consultation, assessment of needs, and education and safety services. As the largest national nonprofit volunteer group dedicated to AD research and education, they can help you locate the best clinicians in your area, as well as gain access to the support networks and resources you need to learn more about your options. Don't let the name of the organization deter you. You don't need to have Alzheimer's disease to make use of their services. Your involvement with them is not proof that you're ultimately going to develop the "disease," nor is it an admission of decrepitude.

The association is run by good, committed local people across the country whose job it is to help you find America's most skilled clinicians. My criticism of the organization is mostly leveled at the administrators in Chicago, Washington, and elsewhere who call for disproportionate funding

> **LOCATING YOUR NEAREST ALZHEIMER'S ASSOCIATION**
>
> There are more than two hundred chapters and two thousand support groups across fifty states. To find your local Alzheimer's Association chapter, go to www.alz.org/findchapter.asp and enter your state and zip code, or call their 24/7 toll-free hotline: 800-272-3900.

for AD lab research over human care. My patients and caregivers often tell me how big a help the AA was in providing the resources and guidance necessary to adapt to their changing circumstances. You should seriously consider utilizing the organization's services. If things work out well, perhaps you can volunteer for them as many former caregivers (and persons with memory problems) have.

> **CHECKLIST FOR FINDING A DOCTOR**
>
> - Understand the options your insurance gives you.
> - Consider your primary-care physician as a first consultation.
> - Use the grassroots approach, seeking word-of-mouth recommendations from others who know of quality specialists in the area.
> - Regardless of whether you receive care from your primary-care physician or a specialist, call or visit the Alzheimer's Association to see how they can help you.

YOUR DOCTOR'S APPOINTMENT

Once you've located a clinician and scheduled an appointment, take some time to prepare for your visit. Anxiety is a normal reaction to the first trip to the doctor's office, but there are ways to mollify it. Knowledge is power. Not only can knowledge about brain aging assuage your fears of the "Alzheimer's disease" myth, but it can empower you to act more confidently in your clinical encounter, to better understand the battery of tests you will receive and the clinical jargon you will hear, and to help you get the most out of your first and subsequent visits. The more knowledge you have, the richer your story will be.

Undertaking background research on your condition—on the Internet or in books like this one—can demystify "Alzheimer's disease" and allow you to hold your own in and out of the clinic. Though not all doctors appreciate their patients bringing information to them (since it takes precious time to read it), I welcome my patients bringing newspaper or magazine clippings. In fact, sometimes their information enables me to do a little research and learn something I otherwise wouldn't have known. Usually, I spend my time correcting the hype from the media that makes its way into our mainstream publications, but sometimes I am handed an article that gives me insight into what a patient's deep-seated concerns or values might be.

Knowledge seeking need not be a solitary activity. Friends and relatives can be helpful throughout the preparation process, especially spouses, who generally know you best. In addition to assisting you to gather information, perform background research, and connect to community resources, they can be sounding boards before your visit, helping you practice what you wish to say to the doctor and talking about how you might respond to what you are told.

Narrative in the clinic

It is helpful if you write down some notes about your symptoms or those of a loved one and highlight the worst that has happened during the course of your or their decline. You should also include a list of all the background information you would like to discuss with your doctor, and compile a list of questions based on your background research that you would like him or her to answer. When my patients bring in a list of concerns to go over in our first visit, it both enriches and streamlines the encounter. Our clinic sends out a form that prompts people to collect this information before they arrive. Because this first visit is the time for the doctor to get to know you, don't expect him or her to draw too many conclusions too quickly. As a clinician, I can more directly respond to the questions and concerns that have been weighing on patients prior to their visit. The most helpful lists will include:

- A chronological synopsis of the frequency and disruptiveness of your symptoms

- A list of the medications you are currently taking

- Previous illnesses, hospitalizations, and surgeries that you've had

- Family history of any diseases, particularly of a neurological, cardiovascular, or psychiatric nature

- Insurance information

- A list of specific questions and concerns

In the past, such assiduous preparation for a visit to the doctor's office may have seemed excessive, but today, such preparation is appreciated. You would be surprised at how many people don't know what medications they are taking. Patients who can share more of their personal stories give their doctors easier access to their world. This exchange of narrative can deepen the relationship and create an environment more conducive to healing.

Establishing your voice in the clinic

After you've done your homework, found a doctor, researched your symptoms and concerns, written down all the relevant information, and practiced your conversation alone or with family members, it's time for you to put it all together in a clinical setting. Some of us have a subtle fear of doctors that lingers from childhood. The clinicians of our youth were stern and seemingly omniscient in their white coats, representing the very essence of authority. When they talked, we listened. When they gave us a pill, we swallowed it (or at least said we did).

Though this antiquated model of the doctor-patient relationship is hard to shake, it is necessary to see in our old age that doctors are human beings just like us. Clinical encounters are no longer monologues, they are dialogues, or even "multi-logues" with several family members, and you, as the patient, must not be afraid to express the type of care you wish to receive. In my experience, having your family with you can be of great benefit. Not only can they share aspects of your story that you may have forgotten to express, they can also take notes or use a tape recorder to assist you in remembering details about what the doctor said.

Different members of the family may have different perspectives to offer. The skillful clinician will incorporate those into the picture he is getting about your situation. The way to do this is to develop a close relationship with your clinician that is based on openness and trust. Such a relationship can enable you to push for clarification, to ask for honest opinions, to raise objections, to disagree. In short, the closer you are with your doctor, the better you will collaborate on telling your story. And the better the story is, the better the care.

> *The competent physician, before he attempts to give medicine to the patient, makes himself acquainted not only with the disease, but also with the habits and constitution of the sick man.*
>
> —CICERO

The most important element of your first visit is to make sure you leave with the doctor knowing your history and details about your current status. Make sure you feel comfortable with him or her, and that your values and preferences will be represented in coming visits. Unfortunately, doctors often make the mistake of ignoring the person with memory problems, particularly if they are severe, and talk only to the family. A good doctor relates to everyone and appropriately makes the patient the center of attention. I usually sit on a stool right in front of the patient and rotate left and right to direct my gaze and attention to the family members who are speaking. If this is not your experience (with or without the stool), you may want to consider looking for another physician. Doctors should not feel affronted if after the first visit you decide that someone else might be better for the long term, nor should you have any compunction about feeling that way.

SELECTING A DOCTOR

How do you know if you have a quality doctor who will provide the care you need? The key is to look for certain cues:

• Does he appear sympathetic to your condition?

• Is she knowledgeable?

• Does he smile, shake hands, and use your name?

- Does she sit at eye level with you and pay equal attention to you and whoever else is with you?

- Does he spend sufficient time with you and show genuine interest?

- Most important, does she listen to you and allow you to tell your story?

If you sense these attributes in your doctor, you are in the company of a skilled clinician who can best assist you in coping with brain aging. If you sense that these attributes are lacking, and leave the appointment feeling that you weren't able to express yourself, you may need to reassess your clinical care.

When it comes to your health, you are in control and it is best to make use of all your resources to find a doctor with whom you can work. The better the understanding between you and your doctor, the more effective you'll be at making good collaborative decisions about your treatment. You must feel empowered to control your own fate as a patient—the worst thing you can do is passively accept unhelpful or uncaring clinical service. *You have a right to choose another doctor if you're not getting along with the current one.*

THE DOCTOR-PATIENT RELATIONSHIP IN THE TWENTY-FIRST CENTURY

As we all know, the doctor-patient relationship has become frayed over the years, and people rightfully sense a malaise within the system that has eroded the respect they feel patients deserve. Our Byzantine health-care system sacrifices patients' interests on the altar of financial return and profit. The solution to this problem is in you, the patient. *In the age of the seven-minute doctor-patient interaction, you need to understand that you employ doctors; that is, your doctor works for you.* You should adopt the mind-set of a wise consumer when you are searching for a doctor, and not settle for a run-of-the-mill clinician who has his or her priorities in the wrong place. The key is to trust your intuition:

- Do you feel you're being listened to?

- Do you feel there is a satisfactory give-and-take?

- Can you continue developing a trusting relationship with your doctor as you age?

THE GOOD DOCTOR

I often say that a good doctor is one who gives you twenty minutes and makes it seem like an hour, while a bad doctor makes ten minutes seem like five. A good doctor should always ask you if you have questions at the very end. Be prepared to take advantage of that, while remaining respectful of the fact that the doctor may have another patient waiting.

WHAT TO EXPECT ON YOUR FIRST VISIT

The following is an example of what your actual clinical experience may look like, but bear in mind that this is based on what happens at my clinic.

Arriving at the clinic

When you enter the clinic, you should expect to be greeted by the doctor's front-office staff members, who will provide you ample paperwork to fill out. Staff members should be amicable and punctual, as the absence of these traits often reflects a dysfunctional office. Make sure you have your medical history and insurance information, along with any other records you feel are relevant to your care. Ideally, medical records should be sent ahead of you. You may be awash in medical forms depending both on what has been done ahead of time and on your insurance plan, but don't be afraid to ask questions: The staff is there to help you.

Once the clinical staff has processed your information, you will be taken into the examining room. Here, a nurse or aide will take your vital

> ### IN THE CLINIC, IT'S UP TO YOU
>
> It is important to remember that you, the patient, are in control of who is in the room with you. If you need a caregiver to be with you, you have the right to say so. And if you wish to be alone (as is sometimes the case with families), that is also your right. Your comfort and peace of mind should be of paramount importance on the first visit.

signs (normally blood pressure, weight, and pulse) and may briefly ask why you've come to the doctor's office. They may also ask you a few questions about any current pain or concerns.

Meeting the doctor

After a short (ideally) while, the doctor will enter and introduce himself. After some social greeting the doctor will often ask you the reason for your visit. We call this eliciting the "chief complaint." At this stage, you, the patient, are in the driver's seat. This is your opportunity to share your concerns and give voice to your cognitive challenges in an open-ended way. Give the doctor the form you have prepared as a reference, making sure

> ### LIFESTYLES OF THE RICH AND FAMOUS
>
> I enjoy caring for a fair number of relatively famous people. Quite frequently, they are the most prepared of all my patients, and will often send along a form ahead of their visit containing basic medical information about themselves. Occasionally, they will offer me an academic CV or a business résumé along with their medical background. Once or twice I have been given newspaper articles about their careers in sports, business, politics, or otherwise. On one occasion, a VIP from Georgia sent me a copy of his biography in the mail before he arrived. I find this preliminary information most interesting, since it provides me— a busy doctor—with a quick and efficient way of getting to know a patient.

that you and whoever else is with you communicate all the essential information. *Remember, the more of your story you share, the better the care.*

Review of systems

Once you've shared your story and asked the necessary questions, the doctor will generally begin by performing an evaluation of your past medical and family history to see what diseases you have in your background. A social history inquiring into your education levels, your religious background, and any bad habits (excess alcohol consumption or behaviors that would put you at risk for particular conditions like HIV/AIDS) often comes next. Occasionally a detailed occupational history might provide clues about exposures to toxins. This information helps us gain further insight into your condition. Next, the doctor will perform what is called a review of systems, in which he will ask you questions about symptoms in different parts of your body. For example, you may be asked about headaches, which could potentially relate to a brain tumor, just as questions about chest pain might help the doctor associate symptoms with heart disease, and joint problems could be linked to arthritis. The review of systems looks for clues in other organ systems that might tip off the cause of your memory problem.

Physical exam

The exam will involve the doctor assessing your heart and lungs and other body systems as part of a general exam. In addition, a neurological exam will be given assessing motor function and sensory perception. Psychological tests will also be administered to gauge your memory, your command of language, and your ability to comprehend the visual world around you. The doctor may ask you to remember some words or remember a list of presidents. He will ask you to follow a set of instructions and to describe the events in your life, to interpret a picture or to draw a picture, or to name common and uncommon objects. Finally, he might examine whether you can imitate hand positions that he holds up. During the entire examination, he will assess whether you appear to be engaged in the task or distracted by depression, anxiety, or other psychiatric symptoms, and will be looking for evidence of small strokes, brain tumors, Parkinson's disease, fluid accumulation on the brain, and other conditions that may impair memory or cognition. Be warned that the doctor will also be looking to see if you behave socially appropriately or not. So if you have a ribald sense of humor, try to button it down on your first visit, even if you are someone who copes with adversity by using humor. However, I should add that in general I encourage humor in my interactions with patients so as to ease tension and facilitate the human dimensions of the interaction.

> *A sense of humor is probably the most important thing you can have when you have Alzheimer's.*[1]
> —PERSON LABELED WITH ALZHEIMER'S DISEASE, TO MY COLLEAGUE ANNE BASTING

I must emphasize again that there are as many ways to do the physical exam as there are doctors, and that your experience may diverge somewhat from what I've laid out. But it is important to at least know the basis by which you'll be assessed.

Mental state examination

Many doctors will ask you to take a more formal structured test of your cognitive functions. One that is commonly used is called a Mini Mental State Examination (MMSE), which is composed of a series of questions and tests that can be assessed on a standard point system. This is not a perfect testing instrument, but it was introduced many years ago and is widely available at most clinics.

MMSE Sample Items

Orientation to Time
"What is the date?"

Registration
"Listen carefully. I am going to say three words. You say them back after I stop.
Ready? Here they are . . .
APPLE (pause), PENNY (pause), TABLE (pause). Now repeat those words back to me." [Repeat up to 5 times, but score only the first trial.]

Naming

"What is this?" [Point to a pencil or pen.]

Reading

"Please read this and do what it says." [Examiner shows words on paper.] "Close your eyes."

Neurological testing

Depending on how your first visit goes, the doctor may end the appointment by asking you to undergo several tests, some of which are CT scans, blood tests, and neuropsychological assessments. These imaging and blood tests are intended to identify what biological processes may be affecting your memory and other thinking abilities. The CT scan can detect tumors, blood clots, or strokes, while blood tests are designed to detect metabolic disturbances or endocrine deficiencies.

Expensive neuroimaging is the latest craze in the Alzheimer's field. Standard CT and MRI scans are a part of routine practice, although there is some controversy about when to use each. However, advanced and expensive neuroimaging techniques have been promoted extensively over the last quarter-century, promising much, but delivering relatively little. Imaging is categorized into two approaches: structural and functional. MRI (magnetic resonance imaging) is a structural approach that provides more details than CT (computerized tomography) scanning, which is the most commonly used and cheapest form of structural imaging. However, these details can at times be more confusing than helpful. MRI scans can show smaller strokes, and that is helpful in the differential diagnosis of vascular dementia; but it also shows what we call "unidentified bright objects," which are of unclear significance and could indicate anything from small strokes, to normal aging, to other phenomena that we don't understand.

PET (positron emission tomography) scanning shows the brain at work, i.e., a form of functional imaging. The most commonly used PET approach traces radioactively labeled glucose that has been introduced into the patient's body. The scanner follows the distribution of this glucose to see which parts of the brain are more active than others. Patients should know that the standard amount of radioactivity is not harmful.

In addition to PET scans, functional MRI (fMRI) scans, which measure blood flow or other dynamic processes, can also be used to study brain function. Unfortunately, the modeling of the living brain is difficult and the images often uncertain in their interpretation, particularly with PET scans. This uncertainty does not prevent many neuroimaging advocates from making exaggerated claims that their particular technique and compound can diagnose a specific condition that was previously thought to be diagnosable only clinically. As a society, we must carefully watch the financial conflicts of interest between neuroimaging companies and their affiliated clinicians. An illustration of this controversy is the use of PET scanning in the differential diagnosis of Alzheimer's disease and frontal lobe dementia. Glucose metabolism is worse in the front of the brain in the latter condition and in the side part of the brain in the former. Yet these conditions often overlap a great deal. Although PET scans can provide some information to assist in the differential diagnosis, most experts, including myself, do not feel that they're useful in most situations. *And* they are expensive. *And* the profits may primarily go to the people who promote their use clinically.

I believe that the clinical history will remain more important in diagnosis than scanning technology, and that we will never have a specific neuroimaging test for Alzheimer's disease. There is too much overlap with normal aging and other conditions. It may be that PET scans of chemicals such as amyloid could be used to track the course of the disease and the effects of specific therapies. However, while this remains an interesting scientific possibility, it remains to be proven. Studies show for example that people with MCI have an amyloid deposition that is intermediate between Alzheimer's and normal aging. Hence, as with many attempts to develop a diagnostic test, the issue is where to draw the line. Moreover, people who advocate for neuroimaging claim that their technology is likely to demonstrate less variability upon repeat testing than a clinical examination with paper and pencil tests. This may yet prove to be true. Yet in their private circles they will admit that we know too little about the reliability of scans across time and place and that pencil and paper tests such as the MMSE are often the more reliable— not to mention cheaper—medium. Despite this, the government is now spending tens of millions of dollars to promote neuroimaging without, in my opinion, a clear likelihood of significant benefit. This is a time in our healthcare system when we should be looking at spending less on a technology rather than more, given other outstanding health priorities. The question we must continue to ask is: Will continuing research into neuroimaging benefit patients or the researchers and their associated companies?

> *What habits, then, might be seen as obstacles to wisdom? Candidates include uncritical acceptance of ideas in vogue, blind following of popular trends of practice without reflection on their merits and implications, the conflation of technological advance with considered understanding of human progress, overuse of technology intended to deflect attention in ever-increasing speed from anything but the content of one's own ideas, pedagogical goals directed at performance to a common standard over encouragement of good reasoning and pertinent interchange.*[2]
> —LISA OSBECK AND DANIEL N. ROBINSON

When decisions are made for you to take medical tests, ask your doctor to explain why it is important, what it will cost, and what the test means in the larger scheme of your health. If you are displeased with what the doctor tells you, it may be prudent to seek a second opinion and discuss your health with another medical professional. If you happen to be in a teaching hospital, doctors-in-training, medical students, interns, residents, or fellows may also examine you. These trainees have a wealth of knowledge and may actually have more time to talk to you. In the case of your health-related decisions, it is best to ask more questions rather than fewer. The better you understand your medical condition and the better your doctor knows you, the stronger and more collaborative your decisions about treatment will be.

A STORY FROM MY PRACTICE

A woman who was active in the Alzheimer's Association once came to see me in a tizzy after researchers in a study had told her that she had Mild Cognitive Impairment. She had volunteered for the study because she was normal and wanted to serve as a control subject (one not in a test group). Much to her surprise, she received a medical checkup and was informed that she was mildly cognitively impaired. As I do with most of my patients, I explained the problematic nature of that label and reassured her that there was a wide range of how memory is affected as we age, and how people's functioning depends largely on how they adapt to the changes. For a second opinion, she went to see a prominent MCI physician at the Mayo Clinic in Minnesota, who also told her that her condition did not warrant an MCI diagnosis, and that in fact the MCI label was in transition. Though comforted by both our words, the woman was troubled by bright objects that appeared on an MRI scan that had been taken at the Mayo Clinic. My colleague assured her that the objects were of unclear significance—"unidentified bright objects" as neurologists call them, which can occur in normal aging, vascular disease, or degenerative disease. On a follow-up visit to me, she told me that while the other clinician had fancier imaging equipment, she felt more comfortable with me because I had the nicer smile! Amidst the extravagant technology we now have in modern medicine, it often strikes me that the most effective therapeutic intervention for those coping with dementia is a caring clinician who will listen.

Second appointment with the doctor

After you've been tested, you will return to the doctor to receive a clinical opinion about your condition. Sometimes more than one clinician may be involved. I call these follow-up meetings "summary conferences," and their purpose is to go over test results and integrate what we've learned into the ongoing story of your brain aging. The doctor will first present the results of his analysis, hopefully in a manner that is lucid, reasonably paced, and free of medical jargon, and then offer recommendations on how to approach it. Besides a rundown of your condition, the doctor or some other member of the health-care team should also discuss the need to plan legal and financial matters like writing advance directives and living wills. Such documents help others in the family make health-care decisions if the patient is incapacitated and unable to decide for themselves. All people regardless of age or medical condition should prepare such documents.

The team should also discuss financial planning such as preparing a regular will and considering insurance needs, including whether to purchase long-term-care insurance.

When the doctor, nurse, or social worker has presented this information, you should ask follow-up questions. It is essential that you turn this into a dialogue and voice your reactions and concerns.

- The doctor may suggest that you begin taking cholinesterase inhibitors, and you should be prepared to ask him or her about the pros and cons.

- Ask about his or her own experience with the medication—both the good and the bad.

- Inquire as to how you can help decide whether the medication is benefiting you.

- Be particularly careful about taking the latest, newly advertised drugs. Such drugs will likely be more expensive, with a less-well-known safety profile.

IF THE MEDICINE'S NOT WORKING

If you do decide to use pills, and if they prove to be ineffectual or if the side effects cause extreme discomfort, make it clear to your doctor that the medicine is not working. Some medicines affect people differently than others; just because a pill is commonly prescribed or advertised on television does not mean it is right for you.

Research participation

The doctor may ask if you would like to participate in research. Research can be a means of helping others and helping yourself, but research studies have some risk. Most research projects require that a percentage of the participants be given a placebo. In such cases, even if you participate in research there is no guarantee that you will receive the experimental treatment or that it will be good for you.

Let's say that this matter of probability does not bother you. Before agreeing to the research protocol you must still have your doctor explain in the clearest language possible the benefits and risks of such research. Some questions you might ask are:

- What is the nature of the pill or other intervention?

- How much do we know about experience with it in animals and people?

- What are the expected side effects?

- If I get sick in the study and the treatment is suspected as the cause, who will be responsible for paying my medical bills?

You should also ask your doctor exactly who is sponsoring the research. Is it the pharmaceutical industry? Remember, you have a right to know as much as you need and want to about the research you are participating in. The basic principle of research ethics is called informed consent. As the potential participant, you, the research subject, need to know what the study is designed to find out and what you will be asked to do. Once you are informed, then you can decide whether or not to give your consent. Also remember that not only must you or a caregiver-proxy-decision-maker provide consent, but also the consent can be withdrawn at any time. The choice is yours to make, not your doctor's. It is noble to want to give yourself to helping others, but you must proceed with due caution and be sure that you are in the driver's seat.

Ultimately, the lesson for the second appointment is to be a strong advocate for yourself or your loved one and to ask the doctor plenty of questions to get all the clarity and explanation you feel you need.

> *I must be one of the victims, I've got a chance to be one of the contributors. I feel quite good about that.*[3]
> —PERSON TAKING PART IN DEMENTIA RESEARCH,
> COMMENTING ON HOW PARTICIPATION IN A DRUG
> TRIAL ENABLED AN OPPORTUNITY FOR ALTRUISM

From the second appointment onward

After the second appointment, you may return either to your primary-care physician or to your neurologist for subsequent visits to follow up on the effects of any treatments or recommendations offered. Often people need time to implement some of the suggestions, particularly as they relate to long-term planning. Follow-up visits can be scheduled for one month, three months, six months, or even a year depending on how quickly one's condition is changing. I see patients more frequently when I am adjusting the doses of medications. However, with responsible patients and caregivers a fair amount can be handled over the phone. A specialist should send a note to the referring physician or others, but should ask your permission to share this information.

FACING THE WORST-CASE SCENARIO

What do you do if you receive a diagnosis of Alzheimer's or MCI on your initial or subsequent visits to the doctor? How do you re-assert your voice and make sure that a standard approach is not used with you? The first thing to do is to keep an open mind, realizing that an AD or MCI diagnosis is controversial and clouded with much uncertainty. Remember: These clinical diagnoses are imprecise and presumptive categories with noncodified classifications, and knowing this is a form of empowerment.

You should raise the issue of diagnostic uncertainty with your clinician and ask him to address the scientific confusion about Alzheimer's and MCI along the continuum of brain aging.

Some questions that you may want to ask:

- What exactly is Alzheimer's/MCI and how is it different from normal aging?

- I've read that every diagnosis of AD is only "probable," so how sure are you that that's what I have?

- I've heard that so-called AD/MCI affects people in quite different ways and that not everyone has the same timetable. Is there hope that my case will be milder than what I read about in the mainstream press?

- Can you imagine a future in which you'll no longer use the term "AD"?

- Can we try a different approach? I'm not comfortable with that label, and I'd like to talk about how we might approach my situation differently.

If your doctor is unable to carry out the type of dialogue that you need, you should consider finding another professional who will be more sympathetic to your perspective. Optimally, you will have already avoided this scenario by screening for a good doctor in the beginning stages of your preparation. Remember that it is your responsibility to be an educated consumer and to seek out a doctor who fills your needs. You hold the power of choice.

CAN THE HEALTH-CARE SYSTEM COPE WITH NUANCE?

I know that de-emphasizing the Alzheimer's label is a complicated endeavor. In today's health-care system, diagnostic labels are necessary for reimbursement. Whether I or other physicians get paid depends on the code that we use: 331.0 (Alzheimer's disease) may pay differently than nonspecific memory loss (780.93). Our dysfunctional health-care system requires that doctors apply arbitrary disease labels in order to get reimbursed. If I could shout this, I would: *We should not let health payers dictate the kinds of stories our medical establishment tells aging individuals and their families!*

I recognize that the medical bureaucracy needs labels. Occasionally a label will get my patients access to services they would not otherwise have, and specific diagnoses will get me paid. Some colleagues have even warned me that patients might sue me for not diagnosing them with AD. But as long as I explain my perspective, and share how I've come to my values and opinions, I believe that I am protected. Besides, the most fail-safe way to avoid lawsuits is to have a good relationship with your patients and their families, and I work hard to develop my relationships, and to serve as a model for doctors in our struggling health-care system.

> **A SUGGESTION TO MY COLLEAGUES**
>
> I encourage physicians who are sympathetic to the ideas in this book to fill in the insurance forms according to the standard Alzheimer's scheme so that patients can be reimbursed. However, this is an entirely separate act from your dealings with the patient and her family. Using standard diagnostic language (despite its uncertainty) on insurance forms is fine; your dialogue with the family allows you the opportunity to address the subtleties of brain aging and approach the labeling process in a respectful and humanitarian manner.

Granted, individual patients vary in the degree to which they will tolerate ambiguity. Some patients and caregivers need labels. Some would be willing to accept that our current understanding of brain aging is limited and be told that they have evidence of age-related cognitive impairment rather than AD. Other patients demand a more precise diagnosis and would become unhappy with a physician unable to accomplish this. Even in individual families, different members will be looking for different answers. My message in this book is not that I have the right story in all cases; rather, I wish to emancipate you and your loved ones from the culturally corrupt myth of AD, so that you can choose to tell the story that best helps you adapt to your brain aging.

A STORY FROM MY CLINIC

One of the aging patients for whom I have cared in the past year, a college professor, was having difficulty organizing his coursework and delivering lectures—symptoms that might otherwise earn him a label of early Alzheimer's disease or another degenerative dementia like frontal lobe dementia or MCI. His partner, also an academic, a historian who was aware of the social and historical context out of which the AD label has emerged, was concerned about his loved one being branded as an Alzheimer's victim. On the other hand, the patient's daughter desired that her father be given a precise label that would do justice to the complex changes that she had witnessed in him. An AD diagnosis might have provided the catharsis she needed to reconcile her father's cognitive decline.

For a clinician, negotiating competing perspectives while trying to do what is best for the patient can be a real trial. I took the time to discuss with everyone the complexity of my patient's condition, and I explained how difficult it was to apply a precise label in his case. They each spoke and expressed how they would like to move forward into the future and eventually came to an agreement on how their loved one would be labeled, which did not involve a degenerative dementia.

Preachers or scientists may generalize, but we know that no generality is possible about those whom we love; not one heaven awaits them, not even one oblivion.
—E. M. FORSTER

HANDLING SIGNIFICANT CHANGES

Over time, as your brain ages, doctors will determine that certain behaviors must be modified. I often ask families about concerns they might have regarding a loved one cooking, as memory loss and ovens can be a deadly combination. Another common point of contention that arises in my clinical visits is whether a patient is able to drive. Someone affected by brain aging may gradually lose his ability to reason and make sound judgments on the road. A person may become lost, respond too slowly to traffic, and initiate or be drawn into accidents. In these situations, it is the social responsibility of friends and family to guide the person to make the right decision to stop driving. Because driving represents independence in our culture, patients understandably resist relinquishing their right to drive. When families urge their aging relatives to get off the road, the disagreements can become acrimonious, and doctors are asked to serve as arbiters.

A STORY FROM MY PRACTICE

One of my patients was an incredibly dynamic elderly man who climbed mountains, traveled the world, and carried himself as if he were twenty-five rather than seventy-five. However, he began to rapidly decline toward the end of his life, becoming socially inappropriate in his manner, and incompetent in his activities of daily living, which included his continued contribution to a legal practice. His children were afraid that his incompetence, combined with his still-present desire to be as active and vital as he was in his youth, could potentially endanger him. They came to me asking how we could help their headstrong father restrict behaviors that could imperil his and others' safety. As I try to do with all my patients, I developed a relationship with the father and ultimately grew close enough that I was able to gain his trust and offer suggestions on what he needed to do to stay safe. In our allied relationship, I empowered him to make decisions on his own behalf, which is always the best outcome for the patient and their family. Good clinicians will realize that everyone including persons with diminished mental faculties can still be included in discussions about significant decisions.

In these situations it is best for the doctor and family not to simply strip away the patient's driving privileges. There is very little that is more humiliating than to have an everyday activity you have performed for your whole life denied to you on the basis of getting older. There are ways to negotiate these difficult decisions in clinical settings so that patients and families can avoid undue strain. For instance, a clinician can raise the question of whether a patient has more trouble driving at night or in inclement weather. If this applies, then perhaps an agreement can be reached about when it is safest for the patient to drive and when it is better to stay off the road. The doctor can write out a prescription to discontinue driving until formal evaluation is completed. A clinician can also serve as a mediator in these debates by recommending that a patient receive a driver evaluation and occupational therapy for driving difficulties. This effectively outsources the opinion about driving ability to a credible expert, who can then make a determination of a person's capacity to remain a driver.

In the event that a loved one simply refuses to stop driving, there are other strategies that can be used to curtail potentially dangerous behavior. Families can hide car keys or disable a car. Some relatives of my patients have asked the police to follow the elderly driver out of the driveway and to write a ticket once any weaving, swerving, or traffic violation is observed. Optimally, the situation won't reach such a desperate point. A good clinician will engage the family and patient in a conversation about driving safety and empower the patient to make his own decision regarding his behavior. If this or any other significant issue is a concern for you as the patient or relative, make sure your doctor knows from the start.

THE WEB IS YOUR FRIEND: EVALUATING WHAT THE DOCTOR TELLS YOU USING THE INTERNET

Computers can be extremely helpful in shaping your experience of brain aging between doctor visits. Everyone has left a doctor's appointment with the feeling of not having received answers to lingering questions. Quite often, the Internet can help you obtain information to fill in these gaps.

A WORLD AT OUR FINGERTIPS

Besides Google and other such search engines, the Alzheimer's Association (www.alz.org), the NIH (www.NIH.gov), ADEAR (www.nia.nih .gov/alzheimers), and Healthwise (www.healthwise.org) contain pages upon pages of helpful information, as well as links to other sites that can inform your understanding of your condition and the treatments and tests you may receive.

Not only can such information clear up misapprehensions you might have, but the process of navigating the Web can also help you stay mentally active. Your use of the Internet need not be purely information-oriented. Reading the stories of others who are undergoing the challenges of brain aging can be a liberating way to see that every experience is a unique one, and that there is more to a sick man or woman than their aging brain. Joining online chat rooms and groups can also provide the opportunity to share your questions and concerns with others who are coping with similar circumstances.

In short, there is no reason not to take advantage of the technology at our fingertips. At the same time, remember that the Web can be confusing and can mislead people in dangerous ways. You should always cross-check information, and confirm information obtained on the Web with trusted friends and authorities.

The Internet is a great asset. Even so, as a medical student at Johns Hopkins, I remember some of the wiser senior clinicians telling me that the most important aspect of medical diagnosis, as well as ensuing care, was listening carefully to the patient's history, to the stories they bring to the clinic. The axiom went that 85 percent of diagnosis was reliant on listening to a patient's story, 10 percent on physical examination, and 5 percent on technology. In other words, the most important aspects of healing were bound up with the human relationship between the healer and patient.

> *Learne thy philosophy exactlie wherein consist*
> *the knowledge of man, the prime subject of medecin.*
> —CODE OF CONDUCT FOR PHYSICIANS STUDYING AT
> OXFORD AND CAMBRIDGE IN THE MIDDLE AGES

Yet in the quarter-century of my clinical career, these percentages almost seem to have been inverted, as an influx of expensive technological equipment, combined with severe constraints on time, has limited the physician's ability to listen deeply to patient stories.

Many people have heard of Dr. Jack Kevorkian, the Michigan doctor who became known by the moniker "Dr. Death" after helping to assist the suicide of several patients. A little-known story is that Dr. Kevorkian's first assisted-suicide patient, Janet Adkins of Portland, Oregon, was a so-called Alzheimer's victim. Her family members said that she had made the decision to die when she was first diagnosed with having AD—that her outlook was so bleak after the brief conversation with her doctor that she couldn't bear the idea of suffering from the dread disease. Even though Mrs. Adkins was still hale enough to beat her sons at tennis, she made the decision in 1990 to contact Dr. Kevorkian and forgo the rest of her life.

Quite simply, situations like the one in which Mrs. Adkins found herself could be managed differently. Brain aging is not a death sentence or a tragic loss of self. And yet, in the note to her family, Mrs. Adkins wrote: "I do not want to put my family or myself through the agony of this terrible disease."

For most clinicians in the aging field, the joy and the challenge of clinical care, and the duty of a good clinician, is to be engaged with patients, to fuse with their story in a healing collaborative relationship. This relationship is what empowers families and individuals to move forward into the future with hope as they face the significant challenges of brain aging. Finding a physician who is interested in guiding you and your family through the brain-aging process, and who has the time and professional commitment to listen to you and appreciate the unique story you bring into his practice, is essential to achieving quality of life at the end of your life. Mrs. Adkins and her family were influenced by the Alzheimer's myth. You must feel empowered to choose a physician who will better help you co-construct the story that you and your loved ones live by throughout your later years.

CHAPTER NINE

A Prescription for Successful Aging Across Your Life Span

Precaution is better than cure.

—Johann Wolfgang von Goethe

My patients sometimes bring me press clippings that range from the sublime to the absurd:

TOWARD IMMORTALITY: THE BENEFITS OF STAYING ACTIVE

BLACK CURRANTS AND BLUEBERRIES MAY
HELP THWART ALZHEIMER'S

MEDITERRANEAN DIET LOOKS GOOD FOR ALZHEIMER'S

FULL SOCIAL LIVES MAY PROTECT AGAINST ALZHEIMER'S

NIH SAYS "USE IT OR LOSE IT"

FISH IS BRAIN FOOD

REGULAR EXERCISE MAY DELAY ALZHEIMER'S

MENTAL GYMNASIUM PROMISES TO KEEP BRAINS FIT

CAMBRIDGE RESEARCHER PREDICTS HUMANS
CAN LIVE FOR 5,000 YEARS

With so many health tips floating around on television, in magazines, and in newspapers, how are we ever to know what is good for us? Are there daily activities that will really help you maintain your brain? Can exercise and diet really enable us to stay cognitively fit? Does stress make the brain age faster? Or is it all just a tease?

Though the complexity of our brains precludes simple answers about the prevention of cognitive decline, I will try to help you sort through these and other such questions. As I've said, any headline promising a miracle cure for Alzheimer's must be read as an exaggeration, and an irresponsible one at that. It is unlikely that there will ever be a panacea for brain aging, and baby boomers should not rely on extraordinary advancements being made in their lifetimes, despite the promises of the AD empire that make their way into our headlines. *Our attention must begin shifting from mythical cure to hard-earned prevention, from expecting a symptomatic treatment for AD to choosing behaviors that may delay the effects of cognitive decline over the course of our lives.*

When we talk about preventing the brain aging of Alzheimer's, we tend to talk only in terms of developing such neuropharmacological products as stem cells, amyloid vaccines, or even futuristic memory-enhancement pills that can treat or perhaps even arrest the most severe symptoms of late-stage memory loss. This is akin to a team falling behind 40–0 in a football game and then opening up its playbook in the final two minutes. As every good coach knows, being successful late in the game requires committed pregame planning that can keep us sharp and poised for the adversity and challenges that lay before us. Aging is a life issue, a several-decades-long process, and prevention is where we must place our energy and our resources. You are never too old to start making better decisions for your brain—and the fact that you've made it to this point in the book means that you are still cognitively vital and capable of making positive decisions in your life and succeeding late in the game!

PREVENTION

A shift toward prevention is desperately needed at this moment in history, as nations must bear the rising health-care costs of increasingly aging populations. In 2005 the annual United Nations report on world population informed us that, globally, the number of persons aged sixty years or over is expected to almost triple, increasing from 672 million in 2005 to nearly 1.9 billion by 2050. Given the modest symptomatic relief of current Alzheimer's drug therapies, consistently disappointing results from recent clinical trials testing new treatment candidates, and uncertainty about the potential merits of future treatments such as stem cells and beta-amyloid vaccines, governments have ample incentive to begin shaping a more nuanced policy that will focus on improving the health of entire populations over their entire life course rather than responding to cognitive decline after the fact.

Prevention is no easy task, and I must stress that by *prevention*, I mean delaying the onset of cognitive decline, or slowing its progression, rather than staving it off entirely. Brain aging is a condition that develops to one extent or another in all of us when genetic predispositions, molecular malfunctions, nutritional habit, subtle injuries, and other chance events interact to bring about adverse outcomes. To extend the metaphor from earlier, aging is not a game that we ever "win"; it is a game we try to stay competitive in. Indeed, there are some risk factors for dementia that we simply have no control over. Age, for instance, is the single most important known risk factor for brain aging, such that the risk of developing so-called Alzheimer's disease doubles every five years after the age of sixty-five. Other studies estimate that more than half the people older than eighty-five have AD, and that persons who are ninety or over have more than twenty-five times the risk of developing dementia than those aged sixty-five to sixty-nine. Bottom line: The older you get, the more likely you are to experience the symptoms of brain aging.

Another risk factor over which we have no control is our genes. As I've mentioned previously, researchers have found that the ApoE-4 gene—which is seen occurring in approximately 40 percent of people diagnosed with AD—as well as other candidate genes, appear to increase risk. Though we can't do much about our tendency to get older or our genetic profile, scientists have identified numerous lifestyle and environmental behaviors and relationships that can fortify us against the normal ravages of age and make a difference in the trajectory of our brain aging.

HUMAN ECOLOGY: A NEW APPROACH
TO PREVENTION

Much past research on Alzheimer's disease prevention has focused only on "end of the game" lifestyle risk factors such as avoiding high blood pressure and high LDL cholesterol as you age. Now we are beginning to expand our gaze and look more ecologically at brain aging, exploring a range of environmental and bio-psychosocial factors across the continuum of one's life—from mother's womb, to early childhood, to adolescence, to adulthood, to old age—that can be modified to hopefully prevent mental dysfunction later in life. This ecological approach considers the complex and diverse bio-psychosocial processes and human-environment relationships that produce the patterns of cognitive decline.

> ### PREVENTION WITH A GRAIN OF SALT
>
> There is no such thing as perfect, incontrovertible evidence for the prevention of brain aging; rarely do we have the luxury of proof when it comes to preventive medicine. As we've all experienced, what is good for you today is often dashed by the study that appears in next week's newspaper. Though the studies I present in this chapter are legitimate and well researched, you should keep in mind my earlier advice to read each study you encounter (especially epidemiological and animal studies) with caution and maintain vigilance against false hope. Despite this disclaimer, I do hope that you will regard this chapter as a repository of "uncommon-commonsense recommendations" that can potentially benefit your cognitive health and the health of your family.

An enriched understanding of the psychosocial processes and ecological relationships that produce the patterns of cognitive decline in our lives can help you act on risk factors for cognitive dysfunction in yourself and in those you love. On a larger scale, an ecological approach can help shift the medical emphasis from symptomatic treatment in the later stages of cognitive disease—which we currently see in pharmaceutical drug development based on the AD myth—to the promotion of earlier, more effective preventive strategies, interventions, and policies that focus on maximizing optimal cognitive development for citizens of all ages. This is an infusion of creative thinking our culture desperately needs.

In *The Myth of Alzheimer's*, we have already begun to rethink our understanding of AD in order to view it as a lifelong process over which the brain ages rather than a late-stage "disease." This chapter will push the new story further by outlining a plan for prevention in the twenty-first century that introduces you to risk factors for brain aging that you can confront to reduce the rate at which your brain ages.

But that is only half the story.

We must not only take responsibility for our own cognitive health, but we owe it to society to take measures to promote widespread cognitive well-being. In addition to offering you a plan for your own brain aging, this chapter makes recommendations for policy-oriented interventions to promote cognitive health on a broader social level. Prevention must become a task in all our lives and a priority for our lawmakers. Baby boomers will not go gently into their elder years and retirement. In fact, we can reinvent both aging and retirement. After all, this was the generation whose activism and energy fed the idealism of the 1960s. If we all take the actions necessary for changing our own lives and advocate for greater societal changes, we can begin to construct a new framework for aging in our culture.

"LET THY FOOD BE THY MEDICINE": CAN BETTER NUTRITION KEEP US VITAL?

This ancient injunction by the Greek father of medicine, Hippocrates, still seems to have commonsensical value today. Since we human beings spend a significant portion of our lives eating, what we put into our bodies as part of our everyday diets is perhaps one of the most important modifiable risk factors we have. It is difficult to draw direct associations between particular foods or nutritional components and the prevention of brain aging. After all, we don't eat foods in isolation, but rather in varying combinations that affect their absorption, and, beyond that, diet is only one aspect of an intricate causal matrix responsible for human health and disease. Even so, a little common sense combined with an awareness of the discoveries made by nutritional science and the insights of ecological medicine can offer you some measure of protection against cognitive decline.

A man may esteem himself happy when that which is his food is also his medicine.

—HENRY DAVID THOREAU

Minimizing red meat and scaling down saturated fats

Population-level research consistently illustrates that one of the most important components of protecting your cognitive health is to avoid a diet high in saturated fats, which tend to increase cholesterol levels in the blood. Diets high in red meat intake and low in fruit and vegetable intake—a consumption pattern common to most of us in the West—have been linked to vascular disease, inflammation, the production of free radicals that may contribute to neurodegeneration, and a diminution of blood supply to the brain.[1]

These trends are not relegated to the West alone. In fact, other multi-country studies that have considered the implications of multiple human diets have confirmed that intake of fat in red meats was the strongest dietary risk factor for Alzheimer's, while consumption of fish such as salmon, tuna, herring, and sardines seemed to reduce the risk.[2] In a study conducted by researchers in Japan who analyzed the food consumption habits of sixty-four Japanese AD patients and eighty age-matched healthy subjects, researchers found that AD patients tended to consume less fish and green-yellow vegetables (containing vitamin C and carotene) while taking in more red meats than controls. The lesson: The weight of most major studies on the dietary aspects of AD seems to suggest that less saturated fats from red meat and greater intake of fish may reduce your risk for cognitive decline. As Thomas Jefferson suggested generations ago, meat should be thought of as a supplementary food rather than as a main dish in our diets, and the meats we do consume should be lean, high in protein, and low in saturated fat.

Thinking like a hunter-gatherer

To understand why such foods as fish, fruits, and vegetables are good for our brains, we need to visualize ourselves along the continuum of human evolution. With the birth of agriculture approximately ten thousand years ago, and the rise of global agribusiness in the last two centuries, contemporary diets have become progressively more divergent from the diets of our hunter-gatherer ancestors who foraged freely for their food. The mismatch between the ancestral genome that we have all inherited (which has been the hallmark of the anatomically modern humans of the last forty to fifty thousand years) and the foods we now put in our bodies as citizens in the twenty-first century may presently be playing a substantial role in the ongoing epidemics of obesity, diabetes, hypertension, atherosclerotic cardiovascular disease, and AD—the so-called Diseases of Civilization.[3] In other words, our bodies and brains have been shaped by the course of evolution to have nutritional requirements that aren't always met by the increasingly unhealthy and less diverse diets of our modern age. Perhaps the gap between our basic biology and modern way of life makes us more susceptible to the major degenerative disorders of our day, including AD.[4]

SOME FACTS ABOUT HUNTER-GATHERERS

- It is theorized that saturated fatty acids provided about 6 percent of the average total energy intake for pre-agricultural humans.

- Both historical and anthropological evidence seems to bear out that the average adult height was substantially higher—nearly six inches—in hunter-gatherer populations (in which the staple foods were lean meats, fruits, and vegetables) than in agricultural societies (in which cereals and starches emerged as the staple foods).

- Among recent hunter-gatherer populations there is an almost total absence of the diseases that afflict so many citizens in developed Western countries. Heart disease, cancer, obesity, diabetes, osteoporosis, and rheumatoid arthritis are very rare among modern hunter-gatherers and generally do not show up until those populations begin to eat Western foods and adopt Western lifestyles.

Such evidence makes compelling the hypothesis that hunter-gatherer diets promoted better nutrition in our pre-agricultural ancestors, and gives us just cause to delve deeper into the implications of a hunting-and-gathering diet compared to our current one.

Imagine, if you can, what the food-finding strategies of our foraging ancestors might be like as compared to our modern-day eating habits. Although the specific diets of hunting-and-gathering peoples would have varied greatly with latitude and season, the daily food-finding behaviors of our Paleolithic ancestors would have generally allowed for an exceptionally wide range of fruits and vegetables with high concentrations of micronutrients and antioxidants. Their hunting-and-gathering behaviors would also have made the meat they consumed far different in composition from the domesticated meats we now consume. Opposite of our grain-fed animals that are high in fat, the meats of our ancestors would have been taken from hunted game that was lean, protein-dense, and low in saturated fats. And since human groups were never far from waterways or coasts, and much migration is likely to have occurred along rivers and coastlines, our ancestors would have had a relatively high intake of fish and other aquatic foods. Archaeological evidence in the form of fish bones and mounds of shellfish found transcontinentally appears to confirm this assumption, and from that we may infer that human biology is well attuned to, and even reliant on, the polyunsaturated fatty acids of the omega-3 (also known as n-3) series fatty acids drawn from aquatic sources and leafy green vegetation (vegetation produces n-3 fatty acids through photosynthesis).[5]

Indeed, n-3 fatty acids are today called essential because human beings cannot produce them on their own and must acquire them from their diets. Our brains are fatty organs, with over 50 percent of their structure being composed of fat, and essential fatty acids such as n-3 fatty acids make up nearly 30 percent of our nerve cell membranes, keeping them elastic and permeable so that electrical signals can pass through with efficiency. In fact, the synaptic junctions where nerve cells connect with one another are made of about 60 percent n-3 fatty acids. In essence, our brains are replenished by the essential n-3 fatty acids we acquire primarily through our consumption of fish, vegetables, nuts, and other foods.

Fish are considered a prime source of n-3 fatty acids because they ingest high levels of algae in their diets, and retain high levels of fatty acids in their skin, which are then appropriated by humans when we ingest fish. This is why many believe that a diet heavy in fish (and in wide varieties of leafy green vegetables) similar to the diet of a significant portion of our ancestors may be neuroprotective, and may also be the reason cohort studies such as those mentioned earlier, which compare groups of people who share a common characteristic or experience over a confined

FISH STUDIES

In a recent study published in the *Archives of Neurology*,[6] researchers followed 899 individuals (average age seventy-six) for nine years, finding that those with the highest levels of an n-3 fatty acid called DHA in their blood plasma were about half as likely to develop dementia as those with lower levels, even after controlling for smoking, diabetes, body mass index, hypertension, and cardiovascular disease. The study was encouraging but should hardly be taken as proof that eating fish oil prevents dementia.

That caveat aside, repeated epidemiological findings associating an increase in n-3 fatty acids with a decrease in mortality, cardiovascular disease, depression, aggression, and dementia do suggest that we should take the consumption of n-3 fatty acids seriously. N-3 fatty acids are sold as over-the-counter supplements in most drugstores, but readers should be aware that excessive ingestion of fish oil supplements has been known to cause bleeding in some people. It is recommended that you obtain your n-3 fatty acids from eating foods that contain the vitamins and minerals necessary to metabolize the fatty acids in your body.

space of time, consistently associate fish consumption with slower cognitive decline.[7]

In addition to its alleged neuroprotection, n-3 fatty acids may have vascular benefits by increasing the dilation of veins and arteries, reducing the viscosity of our blood, and lowering the amounts of fats in the bloodstream. There is some evidence that n-3 fatty acids promote glucose metabolism, and contribute to improvement of mood and the alleviation of joint pain. Unfortunately, since the Industrial Revolution, most Western countries have undergone a transition in the types of fatty acids they consume. Now the consumption of n-3 fatty acids is dwarfed by consumption of n-6 fatty acids, which are found in red meats, and in industrial oils (soya, corn, and sunflower) that are used to make the fried foods, microwave dinners, and snack foods such as chips, fries, cookies, and ice creams that comprise so much of our modern diets.

BEWARE OF TRANS FATS

Statistical correlations have been found between dietary intake of trans fats and occurrence of dementia, while polyunsaturated fats and monosaturated fats of vegetable origin appear to be associated with a reduced risk.[8] Governments are beginning to take action on trans fats, which are mainly produced through a process of hydrogenation (an industrial process whereby oil is heated to a high temperature and treated with hydrogen to improve shelf life of foods) and are present in margarine, vegetable shortening, ice cream, puddings, cakes, biscuits, pizzas, pies, potato chips, doughnuts, and other processed foods. In fall of 2006, New York City banned the city's twenty thousand restaurants from serving food containing more than a minuscule amount of trans fats, and McDonald's has recently pledged to use a trans-fat-free cooking oil nationwide in America. These are certainly positive developments for our hearts and brains.

N-6 fatty acids may be pro-inflammatory and increase serum cholesterol levels that can interfere with neuron signaling. Some believe that the integration of these fatty acids into our brains makes neuronal membranes more rigid, causing signals to pass through less efficiently, and resulting in the inefficient uptake of neurotransmitters such as acetylcholine.[9]

SOURCES OF OMEGA-3 FATTY ACIDS

Foods highest in omega-3 fatty acids are: flax seeds, romaine lettuce, kale, mustard seeds, scallops, cloves, nuts, oregano, salmon, halibut, snapper, shrimp, tuna, cod, soybeans, cauliflower, tofu, squash, broccoli, spinach, collard greens, cabbage, and strawberries.

Consequently, many have proposed that a lifelong diet highly protective against Alzheimer's will have a higher proportion of n-3 fatty acids relative to n-6.[10] This means cutting down your intake of fast foods, fried foods, red meat, and highly processed foods, and opting for a diet richer in fruits and vegetables, unprocessed foods, and fish. All that goes to say that there could be some wisdom in "thinking like a hunter-gatherer" when choosing items to eat, as this would instantly eliminate a wide range of highly processed, inorganic foods with low nutrition profiles and high fat content. While the notion of trying to simulate the diet of our hunter-gatherer ancestors can obviously seem a bit silly on its face, it is a helpful strategy to use when selecting what foods we put in our bodies. While such ideas are speculative, and we do not understand all we need to know about nutrition and metabolism, there is a need to invest research dollars in trying to understand the complex natural systems in which we live rather than in the simple reductionist approaches used to develop drugs.

N-3 SUPPLEMENTS

I love fish. But even so, my wife has been encouraging me to take n-3 fatty acid supplements. I am beginning to do so, but admittedly have trouble remembering to take them each day. I might add that, unlike many of my colleagues, I never took vitamin E, which was all the rage in the 1990s before recently fizzling out in the wake of inconclusive randomized control trials. N-3 fatty acids are being hyped in ways reminiscent of vitamin E, and beta-carotene before it, and oat bran before that. I must emphasize that there is much we don't yet know about the compound, including whether n-3 fatty acids from plants are as good as those from fish, and whether supplements are a help or hindrance. Take your n-3 fatty acids if you wish, but also take care not to overestimate their contribution to your cognitive health until more is known.

The dark side of fish

It does bear mentioning that eating fish to obtain your n-3 fatty acids is a double-edged sword, because the trace toxins that become absorbed in the skin of fish—mercury, PCBs, and arsenic—can do damage to brain membrane and cause nerve damage. While studies have demonstrated that the benefits of eating fish tend to outweigh the risks,[11] it is prudent to consider the type of fish you consume. Conventional wisdom is that larger species of fish such as tuna, king mackerel, shark, or swordfish usually pose a greater threat than smaller species, since toxins accumulate in greater levels the higher you go up the food chain. Currently, the U.S. Food and Drug Administration (FDA) advises pregnant women and children to avoid swordfish, shark, king mackerel, and tilefish and to limit consumption of king crab, snow crab, albacore tuna, and tuna steaks to six ounces or less per week.

> ### LOW-MERCURY FISH
>
> The U.S. Environmental Protection Agency recommends consumption of shrimp, canned light tuna, salmon, pollock, and catfish, which are low in mercury.[12] Herring, sardines, and freshwater trout are thought to have low contamination levels and high n-3 profiles. When preparing fish, be aware that frying can degrade the levels of n-3 fatty acids.

Lessons from the Mediterranean

In recent years, nutritionists have extolled the benefits of what has come to be known as the Mediterranean Diet, which broadly consists of a high intake of fish, fruits and vegetables, legumes, cereals, and olive oil, and a low to moderate intake of dairy products, red meat and poultry, and alcohol. This is a diet thought to be vaguely reminiscent of our hunter-gatherer ancestors (minus dairy, oil, and alcohol), and thus more in accordance with our genetic inheritance.

> ### BENEFITS OF RED WINE
>
> The skin of red grapes contains a compound called resveratrol, which has recently come into vogue. Several studies have shown that this polyphenic compound increases levels of an enzyme—heme oxygenase—that has antioxidant and anti-inflammatory properties and may protect against neuronal cell dysfunction. Red wines are fermented with grape skins, allowing the wine to absorb greater amounts of resveratrol than white wines, which are fermented without grape skins. Thus, some nutritionists are recommending a little red for the head.

The precise amount of wine needed to reap any possible benefits of resveratrol is unknown and will vary depending on your size and weight. As a general rule, you should try to limit yourself to no more than two glasses a night. Recent studies have linked moderate intake of alcohol with a 45 percent less risk of developing dementia.[13] It is believed that moderate consumption of alcohol may protect the brain by inhibiting inflammation and blood clots.

In 2006, 2,258 Medicare recipients in Manhattan not diagnosed with a form of dementia were evaluated over a fourteen-year period. After adjusting for potential confounding factors (age, sex, ethnicity, education, genetic risk factor), the third who were most faithful to the diet were 39 to 40 percent less likely to develop AD than the third who were least faithful, while the third who were moderately compliant were 15 to 21 percent less likely to develop AD.[14] It appears that the various components of the Mediterranean Diet do promote lower inflammation, oxidative stress, and serum protein levels, which in turn lower risk for vascular problems that can contribute to brain aging—hypertension, cardiovascular disease, stroke, dyslipidemia, and diabetes. A diet high in fruits and vegetables will also suffuse bodies with micronutrients and antioxidants that may protect the brain by mopping up free radicals potentially hazardous to neurons.

Was Mom right about fruits and vegetables?

Although most readers probably have heard this ad nauseam throughout their lives, most epidemiological studies demonstrate the importance of fruit and vegetable intake in maintaining brain health. Recently, a six-year study on nearly two thousand Chicago-area men and women showed that on measures of mental sharpness, older people who ate more than two servings of vegetables daily appeared about five years younger at the end of the six-year study than those who ate few or no vegetables. All participants filled out questionnaires about their eating habits and underwent mental function tests that measured both short- and long-term memory over the course of the study. Although everyone declined on their test results over the six years, as one would expect, those who ate more than two vegetable servings a day experienced nearly 40 percent less mental decline than those who ate few or no vegetables. In examining the specific diets of those who stayed healthiest, researchers discovered that diets high in a variety of green leafy vegetables including spinach, kale, and collard greens—which, coincidentally, are most reminiscent of the diet of hunter-gatherers— appeared to offer the most neuroprotection. It is speculated that this protection is conferred because the green leafy vegetables contain high concentrations of n-3 fatty acids and antioxidants such as vitamin E.[15] On its face, this seems to make sense, since antioxidant molecules (which plants naturally produce for protection from the highly reactive oxygen atoms generated through photosynthesis) are thought to neutralize the free radicals in our bodies, which can damage DNA and lead to cell death and tissue damage. Unfortunately, antioxidants only appear to have such an effect when extracted from organic foods as part of our normal diet. Supplements have been shown to be inert, and potentially even damaging. As with n-3 fatty acids, it is recommended that you acquire antioxidants from actual fruits and vegetables rather than through supplemental means.

Spice up your memory?

A recent study of 1,010 elderly Asians not diagnosed with a form of dementia revealed a possible association between curry consumption and increased cognitive performance on the Mini Mental State Examination. The study, undertaken by Dr. Tze-Pin Ng et al. from National University of Singapore, showed that people who consumed curry "occasionally" and "often or very often" had significantly better MMSE scores than did those who "never or rarely" consumed curry.

The neuroprotective effects were attributed to curcumin, the active ingredient in the curry spice turmeric. Like resveratrol in wine, curcumin is a polyphenol that is thought to possess antioxidant, anti-inflammatory, and even anti-amyloid properties. Previous studies in mice have shown that a diet high in curcumin appears to both lower inflammatory agents (cytokines) in the brain and significantly reduce the formation of beta-amyloid protein depositions. Ng and his colleagues suggested that these alleged protective effects can be seen on a societal level, as epidemiological research[16] has shown that the prevalence of AD among India's elderly is nearly four times less than levels in the United States. Although this discrepancy could be ascribed to different diagnostic screening methods in India or other environmental, social, or genetic factors, the findings are nevertheless intriguing. Readers should not, however, view curcumin as a panacea. Its mechanisms of action in the human body are not well understood and some have proposed that it may have carcinogenic properties.[17]

Calorie restriction: Less may be more

Lastly, it is important to alert you to the virtues of moderate eating. Around the world, people from developed and developing countries are facing an obesity epidemic. This epidemic is driven by multiple ecological factors:

- Urbanism
- Expansion of global markets
- Changing family structures
- Changing work environments
- Economic and social stressors
- Spread of the Western media, which encourages consumption
- Increase in portion size
- Pervasiveness of cars and global transportation
- Possible genetic disposition to overconsume

These rising rates of obesity have led to a higher incidence of hypertension, diabetes, stroke, heart disease, kidney failure, and pregnancy complications, and also portend negative consequences for the brain. Human bodies and brains, exposed to seasonal fluctuations in food availability for millions of years, and with genomes shaped by these evolutionary pressures, are simply not adapted to bear the burden of constant calorie overload. Interestingly, studies on calorie restriction in mice, monkeys, and a variety of other species have suggested that a higher intake of daily energy may decrease the life span of neurons in the brain.[18]

Human studies bear out similar results. A recent research study by Giulio Pasinetti et al.[19] found that while high caloric intake based on saturated fat promotes AD-type BAP accumulation, dietary restriction based on reduced carbohydrate intake tends to prevent it. This doesn't mean you should starve yourself, fast on weekends, or cut entire meals out of your diet, but it does offer justification for not eating past the point of satiation, and cutting back on your intake of saturated fats. Eating smaller portions and doing a small bit of snacking between meals may maintain glucose levels in your body that will help keep your mind sharp, and help you avoid binge eating of unhealthy foods at mealtime.

"THE LOOKING-PAST SELF": KEEPING AN EYE OUT FOR OUR LOVED ONES

Beyond changes in our own diet, there are also things we can do as parents and grandparents to ensure a healthy nutritional start for our children and grandchildren. A commitment to laying down a foundation for cognitive health is a gift we can give to future generations. Our prevention can start at pregnancy—one of the most sensitive periods of human neurological growth. Conditions like fetal alcohol syndrome and folic acid deficiency cause changes on the cellular level in developing human beings. Lack of nutrients and other environmental stressors can cause persisting changes in glucose, lipid metabolism, blood pressure, enzymes, vascular structure, hormone levels, and cell receptors, which may adversely affect long-term brain function and expedite its aging.[20]

"Breast is best"

Numerous studies have established consistent and convincing associations between breast-feeding and improved cognitive development and performance later in life. In a longitudinal study of approximately one thousand New Zealanders, researchers found consistent and significant increases in IQ scores, reading comprehension, math ability, and higher exam scores from ages eight to eighteen in children who had been breast-fed.[21] Another study tracked British babies born during a one-week period in 1946 and found that at each subsequent eight-year interval, children who had been breast-fed were associated with better picture intelligence, better math scores, increased nonverbal ability, and sentence completion. Even when adjusting for confounding variables such as socioeconomic status and maternal education that invariably affect the home environment in which a baby is raised, breast-feeding remains associated with significantly higher scores for cognitive development than formula feeding.[22]

Breast-feeding has been considered the healthiest nutritional start for a growing and developing human being. The World Health Organization recommends exclusive breast-feeding for at least six months. Besides the transference of antibodies, brain-friendly choline, growth factors, and hormones, breast-feeding also provides more desirable levels of DHA, an n-3 fatty acid that is essential to the neuronal development of newborns, than infant formula.[23] The presence of DHA directly influences brain biochemistry and functional development, enhancing, in particular, retinal and cortical function. Some researchers have suggested that the very act of breast-feeding may foster cognitive development: that the interaction between mother and infant may trigger hormonal responses that improve bonding and enhance neural growth.[24]

As many mothers and grandmothers know, the breast-milk-versus-formula-feeding debate has been a contentious one since the emergence of the formula industry in the early twentieth century. Aggressive marketing campaigns undertaken by the Nestlé Corporation have been assailed for their role in deterring mothers from breast-feeding, and denying infants its proven benefits. Since being able to breast-feed is a sensitive window of a child's neurological development, health-care professionals who deal with childbirth, especially nurses, must take a proactive role in essential health education. All of us should encourage our loved ones to give their child the best foundation for neurological development by committing to breast-feeding when it is physiologically possible, safe, and feasible. We can also help defend women's rights to nurse their children in public in the name of promoting healthier brains in our younger generations.

A RACE FOR PREVENTION: THE VIRTUES OF EXERCISE

Most of my patients seem to know that they are well served by staying active, and that it is important to develop lifelong habits of exercise. Our evolutionary thinking cap will remind us that before agriculture, hunter-gatherers were mobile and active and may have traveled upward of five to ten miles a day on foot in search of resources.[25] Our bodies are engineered to be on the move, not to live the sedentary lives that so many of us do.

Scientists have demonstrated that physical activity does as much good for our brains as it does for our bodies. It can increase neural blood flow and protect nerve cell circuits that might otherwise be damaged by stroke, diabetes, and cardiovascular disease, enabling our brains to respond quicker to external stimuli. Others believe that exercise activates cellular level mechanisms that improve brain function. Some have found that physical exercise stimulates uptake of neurotrophic insulin-like growth factor 1 (IGF-1) from the bloodstream into specific brain areas, including the hippocampus. What this means is that exercise may enhance the viability of neurons in the brain's memory center and promote the formation of new capillaries in the brain.[26]

HOW MUCH EXERCISE IS ENOUGH?

You need not overexert yourself in the name of physical fitness. Researchers have found that brisk walking (fifteen to thirty minutes a day, three times a week) can improve cardiovascular fitness, which can result in increased function in certain regions of the brain. Stay within a relative range of comfort, and find activities that you enjoy—not ones that you merely endure.

Whatever the case, multiple studies have proven that physical fitness in older adults is associated with decreased incidence of mortality, hypertension, cardiovascular disease, diabetes, depression, falls, and disability.[27] One study has suggested that regular exercise can reduce the risk of AD by up to 50 percent in some people and up to 60 percent in women who have high rates of physical activity.[28] Older adults who have participated in walking programs improve significantly on tests of high-level executive functions such as scheduling, planning, and task-coordination; and studies that have combined light weight training with aerobic activity have yielded even more dramatic results in improved cognitive function. A six-year study published in 2006 tracked 1,700 older persons in Seattle and assessed how their exercise habits correlated with dementia risk. Those who walked at least three times a week proved to be 30 percent less likely to develop dementia over the six-year period than less active individuals.[29]

Perhaps the best exercise is that which combines physical exertion with cognitive and social stimulation. For instance, such activities as dancing, tai chi, and yoga present complex challenges to all participants. Ultimately, these scattered studies can be boiled down to one simple piece of advice: Stay active.

> **BELIEVING IN PREVENTION WITH HEAD AND HEART**
>
> Doctors who work with aging persons have a common phrase: What's good for the heart is good for the head. This means that if you control the same risk factors for heart disease—not smoking, eating right, exercising, and so on—you can also contribute to the wellness of your brain. It's a good two-for-one deal if ever there was one!

In choosing the best activities, a good rule of thumb is to do what you enjoy. Walking and swimming are great forms of exercise that are easy on the body. Light weight training, jogging, aerobics, and organized sports such as golf and softball are excellent, if your body is up to it. Any type of exercise can improve your balance and energy level and can provide psychological and social benefits that contribute to your well-being.

Use your head to save your brain

When exercising, you must be sure to protect against head injury, which increases the risk of accelerated brain aging, especially when there is loss of consciousness or when the injured person is older than seventy. Head injuries at any age can be detrimental to neurons. It is advisable for those who exercise to wear protective headgear or helmets when playing sports and riding bicycles. And it goes without saying that all readers should wear their car safety belts religiously.

Bike helmets are a cheap, simple, and inexpensive way to protect against dementia. Statistics show that the average careful bike rider may still crash about every 4,500 miles, while medical research shows that bike helmets can prevent 85 percent of cyclists' head injuries. Helmets sell in bike shops or by mail order for twenty dollars and up, or in discount stores for less.

When buying a helmet, make sure it fits to get maximum protection. A good fit means level on your head, touching all around, comfortably snug but not tight. The helmet should not move more than about an inch in any direction, and must not pull off no matter how hard you try. For added protection, pick white or a bright color for visibility to be sure that motorists and other cyclists can see you.

AVOIDING ENVIRONMENTAL EXPOSURES

In the December 16, 2006, edition of the British medical journal *The Lancet,* two prominent researchers, Dr. Philippe Grandjean and Philip Landrigan, declared that the role of industrial chemicals in causing neurodevelopmental disorders in human beings represents a "silent pandemic" in modern society. Their message may be a prescient one. Evidence has been mounting that exposure to metals, solvents, and pesticides present in our environment can cause severe clinical neurodevelopmental damage and may be contributing to the prevalence of learning disabilities, sensory deficits, developmental delays, cerebral palsy, autism, attention deficit disorder, hyperactivity disorder, and premature brain aging.

While all of our brains are vulnerable to the toxic effects of industrial chemicals such as lead, methylmercury, polychlorinated biphenyls (PCBs), arsenic, and pesticides, those most susceptible to exposure to these noxious chemicals are children, from the prenatal stage onward. The development of the human brain in utero is an extremely fragile process, as the placenta is not an effective shield against environmental pollutants and the blood-brain barrier (which protects an adult brain from environmental insults) is not completely formed until the beginning of the third trimester. Because the brain continues to develop postnatally and experience periods of high vulnerability, toxic interference at any point of prenatal and early childhood growth can lead to permanent and devastating changes in brain functioning. This early-life interference is often referred to as developmental programming by specialists in the field.[30]

Scientific discoveries about the prevalence of neurotoxic chemicals in our environment are ominous. Perhaps most foreboding is that of the one thousand chemicals that lab studies have shown to cause neurotoxicity, we are only aware of the effects that an estimated two hundred of them have on human beings. That means that there are hundreds of chemicals present in our environment that could be contributing to neurodevelopmental disorders in our children and hastening our own cognitive decline in old age. As the authors of the *Lancet* piece wrote, "The few substances proven to be toxic to human neurodevelopment should . . . be viewed as the tip of a very large iceberg."[31]

Lead

Lead poisoning has contributed to cognitive dysfunction in human populations for at least 2,500 years.[32] Some scholars propose that the decline of the Roman Empire may have been hastened by endemic lead poisoning—a theory supported by archaeological data showing high lead concentrations in the remains of Roman aristocrats who presumably ingested excessive amounts of wine laced with lead and took in lead particles from water pipes.[33]

Today exposure to lead—whether it be in drinking water, in paint, in contaminated dust, or in soil—poses a significant health risk to the neurological development of young children and adults, although adults are more resistant to the effects of poisoning. Lead, a heavy metal, is most toxic to children under six years old, because it is easily absorbed into developing bodies, where it interferes with the growth of the brain and other organs and systems. Research demonstrates that lead poisoning early in life can reduce the birth and survival of new neurons (especially in the hippocampus), shorten the length of dendrites (compromising communication between neurons), and perhaps even alter the expression of genes related to amyloid production.[34] Thus, acute poisoning can cause persisting developmental, learning, and attention problems, as well as hyperactivity, slowed motor coordination, hearing loss, headaches, heightened aggression, impaired memory and language skills, and a lower IQ. The practical consequences of these deficits are self-evident: increased failure in school, elevated dropout rates, diminished economic activity, and increased risk of antisocial or criminal behavior.[35] Current research suggests that the effects of lead exposure on human brain development may be even more damaging than we currently know.[36]

Obviously, public-health policy in every nation must protect children, and resources must be invested to learn more about the effects of lead, help educate families about safe removal of lead from the home, and properly regulate the release of lead into our environment. If I may speak broadly, in most countries, including the United States, public-health policy needs to be developed with social justice in mind, as children from poorer families are more likely to be poisoned than those from higher-income families. In the United States, African-American children in poor areas are also at increased risk, when compared with Hispanic and white children.[37] At our Intergenerational School in Cleveland, we introduced a lead-abatement awareness program in our service learning activities with a learning project involving nursing and medical students. Our students, ages six to fourteen, were educated on how to check their houses for lead and the steps necessary to take if poisoning was identified. You can push for your city or municipality to act on lead poisoning. So take the initiative: Write a letter to the mayor; attend a city hall meeting; search the Internet to learn more about what lead poisoning is and what it does to our brains.

> ### LEAD REMOVAL FROM YOUR HOME
>
> If the source of lead in your home is peeling, chipping, or flaking paint, steps need to be taken to reduce this hazardous condition. The removal process itself can be dangerous, contributing dust with high lead levels. Seek professional help through a lead clinic or government agency.

Methylmercury

Evidence for the neurotoxicity of methylmercury became evident in the mid-twentieth century when researchers observed a rash of spasticity, blindness, and mental retardation in infants born to mothers who had consumed fish from contaminated waters.[38] The U.S. National Academy of Sciences has recently concluded that there is strong evidence for fetal neurotoxicity of methylmercury, even at minimal exposures,[39] and there are efforts worldwide to restrict mercury flux into the environment. As mentioned previously in this chapter, you should take care to consume fish moderately and educate yourself and your family members as to which types of fish retain the most mercury.

Arsenic

Arsenic is present worldwide in drinking water, and there have been documented cases of industrial pollution in several countries. In children, arsenic poisoning can lead to mental retardation, emotional disturbances, and in some cases death, while ingestion of arsenic-contaminated water has long been recognized to cause peripheral neuropathy in adults—

damage to the nerves of the peripheral nervous system.[40] Although the specific relationship between arsenic and dementia is unknown, it goes without saying that researchers should inquire further into its role in neurodegeneration, and that regulatory action should protect developing brains against the ravages of this industrial chemical.

PCBs

PCBs are commercially produced compounds that have long been applied to oils, hydraulic fluids, paints, pesticides, electrical equipment, and other everyday items in our world. Although PCB manufacture has been banned in most nations—including the United States, where Congress regulated PCB production in 1977—they continue to be persistent pollutants in the environment, especially in urban areas. As with the other tip-of-the-iceberg compounds, PCBs are more destructive to the cognitive development of brains in childhood. Pre- and postnatal exposure—the latter experienced largely through the act of breast-feeding—has been associated with lower IQs, delayed developmental milestones, and lack of endurance,[41] as well as impaired motor skills and short-term memory. It is thought that PCBs may also be carcinogenic, and some have suggested that their effects on cognitive development may be masked until adulthood.

Pesticides

In 1962 the naturalist-writer Rachel Carson published the book *Silent Spring,* which is often credited with launching the environmentalist movement in the Western world. Carson enumerated the damaging effects of pesticides in the environment, and galvanized supporters to stand up to the chemical industry. However, today more than six hundred pesticides are registered, and, in the United States, nearly 500 million kilograms are applied yearly.[42] Studies have demonstrated the detrimental effects of pesticides on developing brains. Preschool children from rural communities in the United States have shown poorer performance on motor speed and latency than do those in urban communities where the exposure is less pronounced.[43] In Mexico, children with higher exposure to pesticides had diminished motor skills, short-term memory, hand-eye coordination, and drawing ability than those in urban communities.[44] There has been a linkage between early pesticide exposure and a later loss of dopamine-producing cells in the substantia nigra, a pathology associated with Parkinson's disease.[45]

Ironically, the neurotoxicity of some pesticides is caused by their cholinesterase-inhibiting effects. Recall that current drugs prescribed for Alzheimer's disease inhibit cholinesterase in order to promote increased levels of acetylcholine in the brain. This goes to show how astonishingly delicate a system the human body is, and, further, how challenging it is to develop therapeutic targets that won't disrupt the body's complex systems.

Neurological damage is, in theory, preventable, and this should be one of the paramount goals of public-health protection. When this is considered against the multimillion-dollar race for the cure waged by the Alzheimer's empire, we must demand that our public officials use our resources to further identify the neurotoxicity of industrial chemicals in our food, drinking water, and environment, and that they strictly regulate those with known neurotoxic effects. The "fight" against Alzheimer's disease means avoiding exposures to toxins, and defending our younger generations from the ravages of industrial chemicals on their developing brains.

Why does aluminum have a bad rap?

Other metals such as aluminum have been implicated as risk factors for brain aging, although the role of aluminum in AD is not thought to be causative.[46] Studies going back decades have shown that feeding rats large amounts of aluminum could lead to a type of neurofibrillary tangle. These reports have received ample coverage in the press and given rise to concerns about the safety of the metal. Many patients bring these concerns to my office. What I tell them is that the aluminum hypothesis has been seriously challenged (one might even say totally discredited) and has been marginalized in recent years. When inspected under an electron microscope, the neurofibrillary tangles associated with aluminum appear to be different from those associated with Alzheimer's disease. Scientists have not been able to replicate the findings of increased aluminum in the brains of so-called AD victims. Despite the concern that the initial findings have caused, the whole aluminum theory seems to have been a red herring. As for the population studies that suggested greater risk with aluminum exposure, many other explanations could account for the statistical associations.

Aluminum is a very common metal in our environment. It is present in pots and pans, antacids, and even deodorants. Avoiding exposure would be practically impossible. The weight of evidence suggests that we need take no actions with regard to avoiding exposure to aluminum despite the early observations that have created the considerable consternation and worry that persists today.

STRESS-FREE IS THE WAY TO BE

We all worry that the constant stress in our lives will wear us down. Unfortunately, these concerns are well warranted. Research has shown that chronic stress increases production of the hormone cortisol, which in some animal studies has been shown to accelerate cell death in the frontal lobes, the cerebellum, the basal ganglia, and especially the hippocampus, the neurons of which carry many receptors for cortisol.[47] These damages can lead to decrements in memory and learning.

Obviously, cortisol is a naturally occurring hormone in our bodies, and biological responses to stress may help us cope with emergencies and situations in our daily lives that demand our focus, but over days, weeks, and years, chronic stress responses can prevent us from learning new information (although the biological effects of stress and its impact on memory are not fully understood). In a small clinical trial published in August 2006, Harvard University researchers assigned eight people aged sixty-five to eighty to meditate and do other relaxation exercises for twenty minutes a day. After five weeks, their performance on attention and responsiveness measures improved significantly, while the performance of a similarly sized control group did not.

To avoid stress, you can lower your blood pressure, perhaps through physical exercise and doing hobbies you enjoy. Some of my patients use meditation techniques; others do yoga; still others listen to music or do artwork. I recommend walks outside to nearly everyone. Besides the cardiovascular benefits, connecting with nature can make gentle the constant stressors of our lives. Lastly, try to surround yourself with others who have a calming effect on you and minimize the time you spend with those who get your blood boiling. There is no reason for stress to expedite your brain aging.

We should bear in mind that social environments subjected to material deprivations can reduce individual sense of autonomy, empowerment, and security, predisposing individuals to higher stress levels. As we seek to alleviate our own life stressors we should remember that it is also our responsibility to address the inequalities in our world that place others under chronic stress.

GETTING BY WITH A LITTLE HELP FROM YOUR FRIENDS

Scientists are heralding the discovery of "mirror neurons," a new class of brain cells that may track the emotional flow, movement, and intentions of the person we are with, and induce this perceived state in our own brain by activating it in the same areas that are active in the other person.[48] What this means is that we are physiologically affected by those we spend our time with (not that we needed data about mirror neurons to know that!). So choose your friends wisely, and try to spend time with those who give you a sense of equanimity rather than amplify your stress levels.

BEYOND CROSSWORD PUZZLES: BUILDING UP A COGNITIVE RESERVE

Medical guidelines consistently emphasize the importance of staying cognitively stimulated in one's later years—more commonly expressed in the phrase "Use it or lose it." Doing crossword puzzles and playing cards or chess are often mentioned as offering some protection against brain aging because they help maintain and build neuronal connections in the brain, but cognitive stimulation during your entire life can potentially be a key preventive factor against AD. In a broad sense, *cognitive reserve* refers to the brain's ability to build up resiliency against neurological damage—the capacity of neuronal connections to tolerate a greater amount of brain pathology (BAP plaques and NFT) before you exhibit dementia. Having an enhanced cognitive reserve capacity that the brain can muster in response to damage may alter your neurological adaptive capacity. The mechanisms might include:

- Building a higher synaptic volume of connections between your neurons

- Increasing cerebral blood flow

- Developing resistance to the neurotoxic effects of excess levels of hormones like cortisol and other glucocorticoids

- Promoting resistance against the depletion of neurotransmitters such as acetylcholine and dopamine, which occurs with age

- Recruiting other brain regions to perform tasks

- Increasing cerebral blood flow and metabolism and conferring greater resistance to the neurotoxic effects of environmental toxins

---

A STIMULATING METHOD FOR BUILDING YOUR COGNITIVE RESERVE

A study published by the journal *Psychological Medicine* combined data from 29,000 individuals taken from twenty-two other studies. It found that individuals reporting higher levels of mental stimulation throughout their lives had a 46 percent decreased risk of dementia. The conclusion may seem simplistic, but there is often great wisdom in simplicity. As Leonardo da Vinci once said, "Simplicity is the ultimate sophistication."

The cognitive reserve theory was first developed in the 1980s. In 1988 a study undertaken by pioneering researcher Dr. Robert Katzman and colleagues looked at findings from postmortem examinations on 137 elderly persons and revealed this discrepancy, confirming what researchers such as David Rothschild and others had said years ago, but which had since been forgotten. Besides showing that some brains with high degrees of pathology often exceeding the criteria for AD had very few manifestations of the disease, Katzman's study also demonstrated that these persons had higher brain weights and a greater concentration of neurons as compared to age-matched controls. The most plausible theory seemed to be that some subjects had built up more neuronal connections over the course of their lives, and that their resilience to AD pathology might be said to represent a greater "cognitive reserve."[49] As you know, subsequent studies of nuns and other religious orders, as well as other populations, have continued to demonstrate that plaques and tangles do not equate with clinical dementia.

Animal studies have shown that when adult rats are placed in a complex, stimulating environment they have a higher synaptic density (number of synapses per unit volume of brain tissue) than rats kept alone in individual cages and rats kept with other rats. The lesson these studies have taught us is that the level of stimulation in our environment may potentially build the cognitive reserve for human beings just as it does for rats. Moreover, physical and cognitive exercise opportunities slow the deterioration of animals in a variety of models of human disease, like AD, Huntington's disease, and amyotrophic lateral sclerosis.[50] Despite the results of these studies, remember my earlier caveats that science has not firmly proven the "Use it or lose it" axiom to be an empirical reality, and that animal models are inherently limited. Even so, it seems intuitively true that we will benefit in numerous ways from living an active and engaged life.

The therapeutic power of story

The neurological benefits of narrative (storytelling-based) therapy for those with dementia are becoming increasingly known throughout the field. Since storytelling emerges from memory and imagination, and since narrative springs from an instinctive desire we have to communicate with others, guided reminiscence exercises can stimulate the prefrontal cortical regions of the brain most affected by dementia and directly engage the personhood of affected individuals. In my clinical practice, we are currently assessing whether these narrative-based therapies that facilitate interactive social exchange actually do more to promote quality of life than the drugs we give to our patients. Most assisted-living facilities are starting to integrate narrative therapies into the range of services they provide residents.

One such therapy, called TimeSlips, has been pioneered by Anne Basting, a professor of theater arts and a researcher at the University of Wisconsin–Milwaukee. Anne has recognized that, while a person's memory may degenerate, the human hunger for creative expression never entirely vanishes. Her TimeSlips project, in which volunteers both young and old lead storytelling sessions with older individuals, provides patients the opportunity to celebrate their creative narrative instinct and weave themselves into a multigenerational community through storytelling. As patients peer at ambiguous photographs held in front of them, they are encouraged to respond verbally and emotively to open-ended questions asked by volunteers. While they appraise and interpret the picture, a volunteer transcribes all of the verbalizations into a communal prose poem narrative, which is often vivid and wildly dithyrambic in its nature. The imaginative expression fostered by the TimeSlips narrative therapy grants individuals the enjoyment of agency, selfhood, and creativity once again, and allows them to access and articulate memories that have long eluded them. Even more, by the end of each TimeSlips session, a group of persons with memory challenges has together authored a prose poem that can be enjoyed by others. Anne catalogues these poems online, and has produced an off-Broadway play based on the stories collected from TimeSlips sessions, entitled *Are We More than Memory?*, thereby transferring the stories told to her by people with dementia back into the community at large. Anne has training centers set up regionally in the United States that offer a one-day training in her technique. Learn more by going to www.timeslips.org.

There are other Web sites that capture the power of story for those of us who are aging:

- www.storycorps.net A fascinating initiative that is recording the life histories of our elders and storing them in the Library of Congress.

- www.duplexplanet.com A site designed to portray the stories of elders who are in decline.

- www.memorybridge.org An organization with a mission to foster intergenerational communication and facilitate relationships between younger persons and people with dementia.

- www.storycenter.org A nonprofit organization that assists young people and older adults in using tools of digital media to craft, record, share, and value stories of individuals and communities in ways that improve all our lives.

- www.elderssharethearts.org A Web site that affirms the time-honored role of elders as bearers of history and culture by using the power of the arts to transmit stories and life experiences throughout communities.

Education and the cognitive reserve

Not so surprisingly, the quality and quantity of education we receive as children has been suggested as a predisposing factor for Alzheimer's disease. A study in Shanghai found the risk of developing dementia to be double for those with no education compared with those who had achieved an elementary or middle-school education.[51] Similar results were obtained in a study in Scotland, in which adults with late-onset dementia were found to have had lower childhood mental ability test scores than those in control groups.[52] An analysis of 396 persons who graduated from Cleveland Heights High School in the mid-1940s drew a link between higher IQ scores and activity levels in youth and reduced risk for cognitive impairment in old age.[53]

Though these retrospective studies must be taken with the usual pinch of salt (remember to think ecologically: Many factors in the "causal matrix" other than early education, such as diet or exercise, could have brought about the differences in brain aging), their findings do suggest that the number of years of education may be an important risk factor for brain aging that you can, in part, control, since continuing education—whether it takes place in or outside a classroom—may strengthen your cognitive reserve. Education can increase neuronal complexity and sow the seeds for a lifelong appreciation of learning that may inspire you to engage in reserve-building activities as you age. The longitudinal study of 678 Catholic Sisters of Notre Dame living in Mankato, Minnesota, the Nun Study, demonstrated that women who were college graduates had two to four times the chance of being functionally independent at advanced age than nuns with less education.[54]

When viewed ecologically, the aforementioned studies provide compelling evidence that the trajectory for cognitive decline later in life may be influenced by the amount of education available to children in their formative years. Although it goes without saying, we must all encourage our kids and grandkids to get as much education as they can. An educated brain is potentially a healthier one. Beyond that, the greater the complexity of our mind, the more valuable we may be to society.

LIFETIME LEARNER

At the age of ninety, Elizabeth Eichelaum from the United States became the oldest person to receive a Ph.D. Her degree in education was awarded by the University of Tennessee on May 12, 2000.

I do want to stress that even if you didn't have a high school or college education in your youth, this does not mean that you are doomed to suffer from dementia earlier than others. Our brains are resilient, malleable organs that can be reorganized and rewired at various life stages. Even if you don't have multiple diplomas hanging on your wall, you can still challenge your mind by learning a new language, a new skill, new faces and names, and participating in activities that will build strong neural connections in your brain.

PROTECTING THE BRAINS OF OUR YOUNGER GENERATIONS

Given the effect of education on brain aging, we must all advocate for a more equal distribution of educational resources in the developed and developing world.

Attention must be given to ensuring safe homes for infants and children, since they learn best when they feel safe, protected, nurtured, and in a state of "attentive calm."[55] Children growing up in abusive, neglectful, or war-torn households will have brains adapted to focus more on day-to-day survival rather than developing the neuronal pathways in the higher brain that will promote lifelong learning. Children exposed to abuse or an extreme lack of stimulation may develop cognitive wiring that puts them at a permanent intellectual disadvantage, weakening their cognitive reserve and disposing them to a greater dementia risk in the long term.[56] Again, it is up to our generation—the powerful, innovative, creative, value-oriented baby boomers—to advocate for these changes, to think ecologically and compassionately, and to leave the world a better place than the one we came into.

MAKING A PROFESSION OUT OF PREVENTION

Intellectual stimulation in your professional life and leisure activities can contribute to your cognitive reserve. Several studies have attempted to identify activities with the greatest protective value. Some of my Cleveland colleagues found that the frequent exchanging of ideas and participation in novel activities may result in increased neural activation and mental processing, adding to one's cognitive reserve.[57] Such activities include but certainly are not limited to:

- Learning a new language

- Learning to play an instrument

- Playing board and card games

- Engaging in intellectually stimulating conversation

- Gardening

- Reading intellectually challenging books

- Taking an adult-education class

- Picking up a new skill

- Keeping a notebook or starting an online blog

- Volunteering in your community

- Maintaining a positive outlook on life

ART AS A THERAPEUTIC INTERVENTION

In the building that houses my clinic—Fairhill Center, a converted Merchant Marine hospital—we have art programs for senior citizens. Similar programs exist in communities around the country. Memories in the Making is a national art program that is sponsored by the Alzheimer's Association and hosted in assisted living communities, nursing facilities, and adult day programs throughout the United States. Trained volunteer artists, with help from facility staff, lead aging persons through a one-hour weekly art session. Participants are free to express themselves through painting, which is important if they have lost their ability to communicate verbally. Contact your nearest chapter of the Alzheimer's Association to learn more.

No more bowling alone

The activities in the list above used to come easily to people living in communities. But as Robert Putnam writes in his book *Bowling Alone,* modern societies have trended away from community-based activities and more toward solitary activities.

Studies have shown the deleterious effects of passive-solitary activities on cognitive health. Leisure activities such as watching TV and listening to the radio have been linked to increased mortality in both men and women,[58] while other researchers have demonstrated that the amount of time spent watching television and listening to the radio associated with the onset of dementia.[59] It must be mentioned that certain types of television are better than others. Listening to radio talk shows such as NPR, or to books on tape, and watching the news or educational programming are more beneficial ways to spend your down time—at least I hope so!

A key factor in the benefit you receive is the *type* of programming you choose, which is very much in your control. Studies have investigated the relationship between television viewing in midlife and the development of Alzheimer's disease, finding that, after controlling for age, birth, gender, income, and education, those subjects who developed AD watched an average of thirty minutes a day more television than control subjects, who spent nearly thirty minutes more a day engaged in intellectual and social activities.[60] The key is to watch programs that actively engage your thinking and imagination rather than promote passive entertainment or vegetative habits.

Some activities that potentially detract from cognitive vitality are:

- Watching unstimulating television shows (however you interpret that!)

- Being isolated

- Listening to the radio alone (except NPR!)

- Refusing to challenge your mind with new information and ideas

- Having an incurious, pessimistic outlook on life

- Feeling disempowered, undignified, un-included, bereft of community

THE NEED TO READ

I often joke that patients should seek out a multi-neurotransmitter lexical enhancement device to help prevent their brain aging: a fancy name for a book. Books stimulate many neurons at the same time and improve our access to words and meaning. Some books can leave permanent profound change in our brains and alter our lives in fundamental ways.

A colleague in Britain, Susan Greenfield, nicely describes the benefits of reading in relation to other modern activities: "When you are reading a book, you read it and digest it. You can find yourself staring at a blank wall, thinking about the story and its implications. On-screen stories can mitigate against that. Children are likely to go for the most easily available stimulating things, such as speed, noise and so on, rather than digesting the text. I'm concerned about the effect of all this on attention spans and on our ability to reflect, to absorb information and use it to create abstract ideas independently."[61]

Strength in numbers: The power of community

For decades, social scientists have explored the benefits of social integration. In his writings on suicide, Emil Durkheim observed that participation in community contributed mental, physical, and spiritual benefits.

> *To be fully human is to accept your interdependence as a member of a community.*
> —MORRIE SCHWARTZ, FROM MITCH ALBOM'S
> *TUESDAYS WITH MORRIE*

Since Durkheim's day, there has been a growing body of evidence from literature all over the world demonstrating that social participation and engagement in mentally challenging activities appear to have a positive correlative effect with mental and physical health outcomes, lower mortality rates, lower morbidity, and lower risk of cognitive decline.[62] A 2006 study of eighty-nine octogenarians demonstrated that participants with larger social networks showed negligible effects of age-associated brain damage on cognitive tests, while those with small social networks declined significantly. Differences between the two groups were significant even after researchers adjusted for the possibility that mental decline caused the loss of social connections rather than vice versa. Social relationships offer a multitude of psychosocial benefits, including:

- Availability of emotional support

- A source of information, guidance, and advice

- Diversion from the stresses of life and the day-to-day travails of aging

- Self-esteem

- A sense of coherence, purpose, usefulness, and meaning

- An increased propensity to take care of yourself and seek out professional help

- A sense of intimacy and belonging

- A belief in something beyond oneself

The benefits of social interaction may not be limited to the psychosocial alone, they may also be physiological. Several studies argue that the neural activation derived from basic human-to-human social interaction may help preserve cognition throughout the course of brain aging by fortifying your cognitive reserve.[63] The British academic Michael Marmot performed a study of Japanese migrants to California showing that while diet—particularly the effects of an Americanized diet that raised plasma cholesterol—influenced risk for coronary heart disease rates, the particular protective aspect of Japanese culture that was protective was the degree to which people remained in the confines of their ethnic group.[64] A caring community can be protective and health-promoting; social environment matters.

> **THE ELDERCARE LOCATOR**
>
> Community organizations are offering programs that stimulate thought, discussion, and personal connections. Your local elder-care agency may know of one. Call Eldercare Locator at 1-800-677-1116 or visit www.eldercare.gov.

Numerous studies have considered the specific types of social interactions and social relationships that are most beneficial. One study following a population of women in Tecumseh, Michigan, from 1967 to 1979 found that the frequency of church attendance was inversely related to mortality and dementia even after other potentially confounding factors such as health, financial status, and gender were controlled for.[65]

Similarly, a study undertaken in Alameda County in California found an association between a reduced risk of mortality and a strong marriage, close contact with friends and relatives, church attendance, and membership in nonchurch organizations.[66] Those most isolated were prone to cognitive deterioration, even after controlling for measures of physical health. Like Marmot's study, these results seem to suggest that regular participation in structured social activities, as well as membership in social networks, have physiological benefits, and that various forms of community involvement can be protective against brain aging.

Interestingly, research has also linked volunteerism with improved cognitive health outcomes and overall mortality. Why might this be? Obviously, health is dependent in part on one's relationships with others, and relationships created by such activities as volunteering offer a multitude of psychosocial benefits, including: providing a means of coping with health changes, improving quality of life, reducing depressive symptoms, anxiety, and stress, providing feelings of usefulness, growth, fulfillment, and self-respect, and protecting against role loss and social isolation. It is also speculated that the protective effect of social participation is derived from the support conferred by human communities.

Persons who volunteer and interact with others in a community setting are also challenged in their abilities and competencies, and the influence of this challenge is stimulating on the cellular level. For instance, depression and stress are frequently associated with chronic medical illnesses later in life such as cardiovascular disease and have been linked to increased platelet activation, undernutrition, poor immune response, and increased levels of the cytokine interleukin-6, and stress hormones (glucocorticoids such as cortisol, and norepinephrines)—all of which are associated with poor cognitive and functional outcomes. Additionally, magnetic resonance imaging of depressed patients has revealed structural abnormalities in areas related to the cortical-striatal-pallidal-thalamus-cortical pathway, including the frontal lobes, caudate, and putamen,[67] and recent research has demonstrated a smaller hippocampal volume in depressed elders who develop dementia over time.[68]

Taken together, the lesson from these studies is: Get out into your community; try a new social activity or skill you've never done before. Encourage your aging parents and relatives, as well as your iPod-listening, Xbox-playing kids, to do the same. Find out what your town or municipality offers and contribute to it. No more bowling alone!

Let's rediscover the unity in community

In the twenty-first century—an age in which we are increasingly connected by cell phones, e-mail, and instant messaging, but paradoxically drawn further apart by quick and impersonal exchange—there is a great need to reengage with our communities to overcome the isolating effect such technology has had on all of us. *Investing time in your community* not only builds your cognitive reserve, it also builds social capital that benefits us all.

Health care will also find a more fruitful future by reembracing the myriad benefits of community. All over the world, healing is an activity undertaken in social settings. It is only in Western biomedicine that healing is assumed to take place solely in the solitary interaction between a doctor and a patient. Our health-care system is predicated on this notion, which has, quite ironically, led to the depersonalization of care. As a society, we must recognize the potential for healing that exists in interactions between fellow human beings, and begin building opportunities for community-level healing into our mainstream provision of health care. The building in which my practice is housed in Cleveland provides a good model of how health-care institutions of the future might integrate better with society. In several acres of space, we have a memory and aging clinic, an intergenerational school where aging persons can volunteer, art therapy classes, adult education courses, computer classes, and the offices of several organizations such as the Alzheimer's Association and local hospice facilities. This sort of arrangement assembles many important community organizations that meet the multiple needs of aging persons and their families. We often hear that it takes a village to raise a child; well, it also takes a village to help persons age with dignity.

THE BOUNDARIES OF COMMUNITY

I feel obliged to say that social engagement is not a universal criterion for cognitive wellness. Indeed, many studies on successful aging have found that some older adults may exhibit adaptive, healthy aging because they reduce social interaction in their lives and thus avoid the stress and strain it can cause.[69] Successful aging is not prescriptive; it occurs on a case-by-case basis. Ultimately, you need to assess your own life domain and make the decisions that you feel will best promote your wellness.

Can the workplace promote the cognitive health of baby boomers?

Most jobs require us to have social interactions and to use our minds in challenging situations, and can compel us to be physically active, punctual, and driven by a daily sense of purpose. These benefits are positive in the face of the fact that there is little chance of baby boomers retiring as their parents did. Working into old age may now be a financial necessity or a personal choice for our generation. Whatever the case may be, work has the potential to be protective for individuals and good for society as a whole. Maintaining the presence of elders in the workplace can be a tremendous boon to businesses and organizations. Elders are known for their work ethic and integrity, and aging persons possess wisdom and an ability to see the big picture. If a job needs sharp, quick thinking and retrieval of new names, words, and facts—what we call "fluid intelligence"[70]—then youth prevails. But if a task requires wealth of knowledge, experience, commitment, and broad vision—so-called crystallized intelligence[71]—then elders are well positioned to contribute.

A STORY FROM MY PRACTICE

I once had a patient who had been a partner at an international law firm. We did preliminary testing on him and it was determined that he had a slight frontal lobe vascular lesion, and some executive functioning difficulties. Even so, I encouraged him not to let the dementia deter him from living his life and giving back to his community. And sure enough he has since stayed very much in the public realm, helping innovate local schools, serving on boards for social organizations, and even teaching in public schools. Here is an example of a man who could've dropped out after his diagnosis but ended up doing just the opposite.

By 2015 nearly one-third of the total U.S. workforce will be fifty or older, up from 27 percent in 2005.[72] As the proportion of younger workers continues to decline, it will become critical for employers who seek to retain a competitive edge in the marketplace to retain and attract older workers. There are strategies employers can use to do so. As the first boomers begin to head into their sixties, some companies are making sure they hang onto their workers by offering flex time, extra benefits, and paid family leave so that employees can handle their personal issues, including taking care of aging parents of their own.

Other companies have been creative in allowing seasonal employment, so that workers may spend the winter months in a warmer part of the country and work from long distance. Admittedly, the working world can be quite harsh to aging people. Businesses are getting rid of many aging workers who have big salaries, long vacations, and accrued benefits. But aging workers are not simply a drag on a company's bottom line: Their "crystallized intelligence" can be an invaluable asset. Creative employers can develop strategies to maximize the productivity of their aging workforce, and tap into the cognitive advantages, wisdom, and know-how of older workers.

What aging persons bring to the world

Potential Disadvantages Compared to Youth

- Slower at learning new facts

- Slower retrieval of names and words

- Difficulty recalling events with clarity

Potential Advantages Over Youth

- Ability to place information in a meaningful context

- Ability to use a great number of words in more novel ways

- Ability to use memory of life situations to draw general conclusions (which we might refer to as "wisdom")

- Supervisory skills

- Ability to track others' intentions and read people's motives

- Strategic, long-term-oriented thinking

- More patient and tolerant of others; better able to facilitate discussions

- A repository of cultural, historical, and personal information

---

LET'S GIVE OUR KIDS THE BEST CHANCE WE CAN

Early-childhood development illustrates the importance of home environments in facilitating a social sense that involves an awareness of oneself in relation to others and an ability to empathize with the emotions of others. Prolonged trauma in early life can interfere with the development of brain systems, resulting in extreme anxiety, depression, and difficulty forming attachments to others.[73]

We need to advocate for the allocation of funding for programs that promote prevention of child abuse, early intervention for abused children, and healthy childhood development, as well as programs that cultivate parental nurturing skills, including home visitation programs that provide services to at-risk families before and after the birth of children. We must also commit resources for community programs and public spaces that offer children, adults, and the elderly an opportunity to read, think, discuss, interact, and learn new things at any stage of their life.

JOINING THE GLOBAL FIGHT AGAINST INFECTIONS

Research has linked early-childhood infections to various forms of damage, including chronic inflammation, that may contribute to aging and mortality. Although causal links between the acute illnesses earlier in life and aging have not been well established, it is clear that bacteria, viruses, parasites, and other infectious agents can impair the neurodevelopment of children. Infections like tuberculosis, diarrhea, parasite-borne diseases like malaria, periodontal disease, and bacterial infections—all of which occur with the highest frequency in impoverished parts of the developing world—raise levels of inflammatory proteins, including C-reactive protein (CRP), interleukin-6, tumor necrosis factor (TNF), and fibronigen protein. Though these proteins are adaptive responses to infections or internal injury in the short term and help our bodies regain health, the continued presence of these proteins in the bloodstream may lead to chronic inflammation that can cause profound vascular damage and precipitate the development of Alzheimer-like symptoms.[74]

Additionally, other studies have shown that bodies are placed under severe oxidative stress when they must continually fight infections. The free radicals and aflatoxins produced by inflammation can damage neurons and other cells, expediting the onset of neuronal death seen in dementia.[75]

There emerges an obvious need to protect against early-childhood infections in our own lives, with children and grandchildren, and in the developed and developing world. This means not only increasing efforts to fight infectious diseases, but also redoubling efforts to combat famine, because infection and malnutrition are part of a vicious circle in which infection can precipitate malnutrition by affecting the absorption of nutrients and the depletion of nutrients can cause further infection. Bill and Melinda Gates, two fellow boomers, have made the fight against infectious diseases the primary focus of their philanthropy for a reason: It is one of the most important global issues that our generation must address.

Taking on global warming

Addressing the challenge of infectious diseases also means taking action against global warming. Elevated temperatures may increase the number and distribution of insects such as mosquitoes that carry diseases like malaria; may promote bacterial growth leading to greater risk of food poisoning and diarrheal disease; and may warm waters and promote flooding, amplifying the risk of waterborne infections such as cholera. Moreover, aging persons are disproportionately affected by drastic changes in temperature, as has been evidenced by high mortality rates during severe heat waves in several countries.

As Al Gore and others have taught us, we can all make small changes in our lives to combat global warming by:

- Recycling

- Driving less and walking more

- Carpooling or taking public transportation

- Flying less

- Reducing our reliance on air-conditioning and heating

- Using energy-efficient products

- Choosing green energy for our homes

- Supporting public efforts to pursue alternative sources of energy

- Supporting local and national politicians who will take measures against the warming of our world

PREVENTION IS KEY

John Knowles, the former president of the Rockefeller Foundation, once predicted that "the next major advance in the health of the American people will be determined by what the individual is willing to do for himself." At this moment in history, our attention must begin shifting in earnest from cure to prevention, from expecting a symptomatic treatment for a "disease" called Alzheimer's to choosing behaviors, and advocating and voting for policies that may be able to delay the effects of cognitive decline over the course of our lives.

There's still time for all of us to make changes in our lives, and in the lives of our family members and our communities, to promote healthy brain aging. I have shared several behavioral modifications you can make in your life to promote your own cognitive wellness and several strategies you can use to think more ecologically about brain aging. Although eating well, exercising, reducing stress, limiting exposure to neurotoxic substances, building a cognitive reserve, and fighting infectious diseases can enable us to live healthier lives, I cannot emphasize enough the therapeutic benefit gained by maintaining an active engagement in your community and advocating for social justice issues that you believe in. This, above all, is a significant intervention we have against brain aging, and is something over which we all have a large degree of control.

> The Japanese have a term that is central to their conceptions of positive aging called *ikegai*. This word implies a sense of happiness found in having a purpose in life. Purpose and selfhood are often found embedded in family and community.

A plan for prevention

Diet

- Eat fewer saturated and trans fats and fast and processed foods.

- Eat more fish and healthy fats (omega-3).

- Eat more fruits and vegetables (vitamins and minerals, antioxidants).

- Lower sodium intake.

- Restrict your daily calories.

- Enjoy alcohol in moderation.

Protecting Young Minds

- Promote breast-feeding in your family.

- Support the right of women to breast-feed in public.

- Ensure that all children are able to eat nutritious diets in their formative years.

Exercise

- Elevate your heart rate fifteen to thirty minutes a day, three times a week.

- Pick activities you enjoy.

- Protect your brain when exercising.

Environmental Exposures

- Limit consumption of fish known to be major carriers of toxins.

- Make your house free of lead and other toxins.

- Advocate locally for lead-abatement programs and attention to other environmental toxins.

Stress

- Exercise and participate in stress-relieving hobbies.

- Surround yourself with persons who calm you.

Building a Cognitive Reserve

- Engage in stimulating activities.

- Get all the education you can.

- Learn new skills.

- Advocate for a more equitable distribution of resources in our schools.

Staying Vital in Your Later Years

- Don't be afraid to seek help from doctors and other health-care professionals.

- Choose a job that stimulates you.

- Learn a new language.

- Learn to play an instrument.

- Play games/cards with a social group.

- Engage in intellectually stimulating conversation.

- Tend a garden.

- Read intellectually challenging books.

- Take an adult-education class.

- Volunteer in your community.

- Maintain a positive outlook on life.

- Advocate for your beliefs.

Protecting Against Infections

- Avoid infections in early childhood and maintain good health care for yourself and your family.

- Contribute to the global fight against infectious diseases.

- Choose behaviors that protect against global warming.

EPILOGUE

THINKING LIKE A MOUNTAIN:
THE FUTURE OF AGING

The world revolves, not around the creators of new noises, but the creators of new values.

—FRIEDRICH NIETZSCHE

One of my favorite things to do is to hike in the mountains, which have long served as a source of inspiration to mankind. While visiting Oslo, Norway, in 2006, I sought out a ninety-year-old philosopher named Arne Naess, a colorful character who lived part of the year in a shack nestled in the mountains. At age twenty-seven, he had become the youngest professor at the University of Oslo and there coined the term "deep ecology" to express the idea that human beings are intimately and spiritually connected to the earth. Though he was affected by dementia, Arne was still a fount of wisdom when we met. As we sat in a restaurant overlooking Oslo, he emphasized a truism that he lived by: "Think like a mountain."

At first this notion perplexed me, but as I thought about it, the metaphor made sense and I began to understand what Arne had meant about the wisdom of mountains. Their weathered surfaces convey a sense of slow change that reflects the natural processes of our own aging. Their peaks and summits inspire us to elevate our thinking, while their wide foundations remind us of the virtues of being well grounded. Perhaps most important, in the ancient ecosystems of mountains we also see the need for our species to keep adapting as we move into the future. But what humans have over mountains is our creativity, ingenuity, and agency—the capacity to influence our environment and take some control of our own aging process.

Ever so slowly, the landscape of aging is evolving. As we embark on the path of our own brain aging—individually and collectively—we must look ahead to the changes that await us so that we can best adapt. The preceding chapters have laid a foundation for the emergence of a new story of brain aging. Now I would like to reach higher and share with you some of the loftier goals and visions I have for the future of aging.

PEAK 1: CLIMBING THE SLOPE
OF OUR DEATH ANXIETY

As it does for many human beings, the concept of death evokes both anxiety and resolve in me. Anxiety because death is the ultimate unknown; resolve because finitude can be the greatest benefactor of the life we lead on earth. Steve Jobs, the CEO of Apple and a cancer survivor, put it most eloquently in a graduation speech given at Stanford in 2005. He said, "No one wants to die. Even people who want to go to heaven don't want to die to get there. And yet death is the destination we all share. No one has ever escaped it. And that is as it should be, because Death is very likely the single best invention of Life."[1]

There is great wisdom in these words.

> *Every day, therefore, should be regulated as if it were the one that brings up the rear, the one that rounds out and completes our lives.*
>
> —SENECA

Baby boomers have been conditioned to regard death with fear—to turn away from our mortality. We elevate to the top of the best-seller list those books that promise to help us live longer, and have created a thriving industry out of products that make us look a couple of years younger. We place ourselves on diets that promise to tack on years to our life, and undergo medical procedures that will help us live longer. Although the instinct for survival is a powerful driving force intrinsic to all human beings, our culture does little to encourage our deep reflection about the precious little time we have on earth, and to help us draw inspiration from our mortality.

Death, or at least the process of dying, can be terrifying, but the confines it places on all of our lives should endow each of us with an awesome sense of vitality and urgency. Without the finitudes and limits of our embodiment, life might well be bereft of purpose and meaning. In Jonathan Swift's *Gulliver's Travels*, the main character, Gulliver, hears about a race of immortal people called Struldbruggs. While Gulliver's reaction is at first one of envy, he soon learns that the reality of life as a Struldbrugg is not so desirable, and that the prospect of never dying is actually a most dreadful fate. We learn that, as a result of their condition, the Struldbruggs "were not only opinionative, peevish, covetous, morose, vain, [and] talkative, but uncapable of friendship, and dead to all natural affection, which never descended below their grand-children." The Struldbruggs longed for death and lamented the meaninglessness and waywardness of their lives precisely because they knew that *accepting our limitations and facing our inevitable death will imbue our lives with meaning, strength, and purpose.*

> *The fear of death follows from the fear of life. A man who lives fully is prepared to die at any time.*
> —MARK TWAIN

> *Look not mournfully into the past. It comes not back again. Wisely improve the present. It is thine. Go forth to meet the shadowy future, without fear.*
> —HENRY WADSWORTH LONGFELLOW

This generative potential can motivate baby boomers into becoming agents of great change in the world. Once we abandon the old myths we have inherited that depict old age as a descent into an abyss of hopelessness, frailty, and mental lethargy, we can begin to view aging as a dynamic process of personal transformation in a new life stage. Some neurosis will likely always surround our mortality. We can either choose to let this neurosis terrify us or put it to work for us and let it motivate us to:

- Treat our loved ones better

- Reaffirm our relationships with those who give our lives meaning

- Take better care of our bodies and minds

- Protect the bodies and minds of younger generations

- Truly stand for what we believe in

- Take creative risks

- Develop new skills

- Leave the earth knowing that we've made our communities a better place and left the world in better condition for our children and grandchildren

- Take an interest in the growth and development of other (younger) people

- Travel

- Gain new experiences

- Seek wisdom in ourselves and in others

BACK TO SOCRATES

I began an earlier chapter with a story about Socrates standing at the gates of Athens. Equally compelling is the story of the philosopher's death. As Socrates lay dying on his bed after being unjustly ordered to death by the Athenian court, he issued a final instruction to his disciples, telling them that they should "practice dying." Socrates' wisdom was that it is not until we accept our mortality that we truly begin to live. And to live means to stay cognitively vital, to have a purpose greater than ourselves, to recognize our embeddedness in local communities and in the broader community of humanity, to take responsibility for the environment that we collectively share, to accept that our legacy is to leave a better world for our children and grandchildren. *To "practice dying" is to succeed in living.*

Ending the myth of Alzheimer's is not just about putting closure to a singular disease. It is an invitation to think more deeply about what it means to be a mortal human being who ultimately ages and exits this life. If we who are aging can project ourselves into a different story, and develop new visions and goals for ourselves and for society, "ending Alzheimer's" can be a gateway to a more meaningful future.

- Be a lifelong learner

- Make every moment of our lives matter

> *To fear death, gentlemen, is no other than to think oneself wise when one is not, to think one knows what one does not know. No one knows whether death may not be the greatest of all blessings for a man, yet men fear it as if they knew that is the greatest of evils. And surely it is the most blameworthy ignorance to believe that one knows what one does not know.*
>
> —PLATO

An exercise in embracing mortality: The LifeBook approach

In my clinic, we have developed several narrative interventions to help my patients reflect on end-of-life issues. One is a project called LifeBook, which is a scrapbook that my patients put together to accomplish three goals:

- Tell the story of their life

- Envision what they want their end-of-life care to be

- Reflect on their legacy

The questions I ask my patients when we are putting together a LifeBook identify their specific needs, desires, habits, values, beliefs, and preferences that can guide future caregivers in managing their daily care.

Pictures, written and spoken narratives, and letters with a strong stamp of personhood are integrated into a book that can potentially assist caretakers in making decisions most consistent with individual values in times of medical need. At the end of the book are placed ethical wills and advance directives to guide decision making near the end of life. Creating a document that so uniquely characterizes them can assure that their final years are lived with self-respect, dignity, and quality of life.

A scrapbook such as this is easily transportable and can be turned to if and when you or a loved one begins to decline, loses ability to make decisions, or in the event that a move must be made to another residence such as a long-term-care facility. Not only can it be an important repository of a person's values and goals for end-of-life care, it can serve as an artifact of a person's legacy after they've passed away. The main lesson of LifeBook is that it behooves you to think more deeply about the life you have lived and how you want that life to come to an end. And the best thing about LifeBook is that anyone can make one—all you need is a scrapbook and a few supplies. Here are several activities that can help you begin to think about the important questions surrounding your end-of-life care:

- Gather pictures of the most important people in your life, particularly those you might ask to help you make important decisions about your future medical care. Place them in your LifeBook and write about what each person means to you. To whom would you entrust your decision making at the end of your life?

- Imagine that you were asked to live in another state and had only one suitcase to transport your possessions from your home. What ten to fifteen most cherished objects would you choose to take with you? Write a few sentences about why each object is important to you. If possible, take pictures of these possessions and include them in your scrapbook.

- Reflect on the questions below and record your answers either in writing or with an electronic recorder:

  - How was your name chosen?

  - Can you recall your very first memory?

  - Can you describe what your parents were like? What about your grandparents?

  - Did you have any special pets?

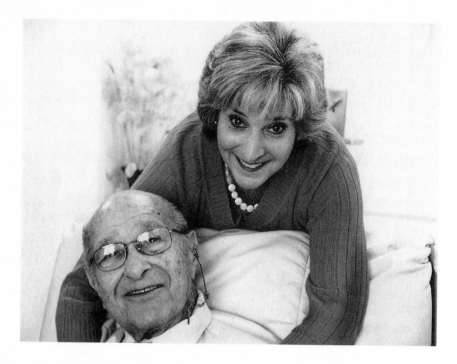

Figures 11A and 11B. Sharing a Multimedia Life Story   Two of my patients, Helen and Milton Krantz, participated actively in many of our local educational and research programs. Helen's memory problems were due to a combination of aging and concern about her husband Milton's more severe memory problems. Milton is seen in the photo above with his daughter, Ellen, whose love and affection helped her parents do so well in their later years.

- If you are/were married, how did you meet your partner(s) and what was your courtship like?

- If you have children, can you describe their birth, or any key memories you have of them?

- What do you consider your greatest accomplishment in life?

- Have there been any particularly powerful spiritual moments in your life?

- What is your favorite book, movie, holiday, vacation, family tradition, music, hobby?

- If you were ever unable to make decisions for yourself, what would it be most important for your caregiver(s) to know about you?

- For what in your life are you most grateful?

- Imagine that you're sitting down to the perfect meal: What's on the table?

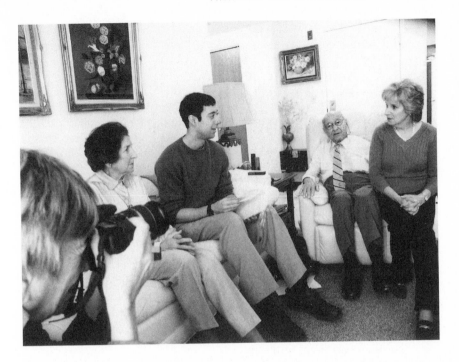

In this photograph, Cathy Greenblatt, a visual sociologist and author of *Alive with Alzheimer's*, is photographing Helen, Milton, and Ellen as they participate in a multimedia intergenerational narrative project in their apartment. Ellen helped Helen prepare her LifeBook for the inaugural project described in the text. The Krantzes were alive with story and hence alive as human beings in the community. (Photos courtesy of Peter Whitehouse)

- What are the most important life lessons you've learned? When you think about what you want to be remembered for, what do you wish to hand down to others so that they might learn and benefit from the life you've lived?

- What are the core values you've tried to live by?

- Compose a short letter to a relative—perhaps a grandchild, born or unborn—who will follow you in the future. Think ahead fifty to a hundred years: What wisdom would you wish to impart to your relatives? How would you like to live on in their eyes? What would you like them to learn from your life? What is the one thing you want to tell them about the life you lived?

- Compose a brief letter to your doctor/caregiver. Imagine that you can't express yourself clearly at the end of your life. What would you want the people who will be responsible for your medical care to know about you? In caring for you, what personal information is it most important for them to consider?

- How would you like to be treated if you increasingly suffered from the symptoms of dementia?

- At what point does your quality of life dictate that doctors should not keep you alive?

- Whom do you most trust to make decisions on your behalf?

- Would you want specific provisions made so that you spend the end of your life at home, or in hospice care?

- All people—young and old—should have a document to guide their health care if they become incapacitated and unable to make decisions for themselves. These documents are called living wills or advance directives. If you have an advance directive that informs others of your plan for future medical care, you may wish to include it in your scrapbook. If not, you should ask your doctor, lawyer, and family to help you create one.

- Assemble any other documents that may be relevant to your future care. For example:

- Do you have any requests for your funeral plans?

- Do you have any specific requests to your family or your main caregivers in time of illness and death?

- If you were in attendance for your own funeral, what would you want those speaking to say? Write a letter expressing what would make you most happy to hear from your family and friends.

Embracing hospice care

Everyone fears that life will end with them hooked up to machines in a cold, sterile hospital, or in a threatening, unfamiliar facility far from home. Despite the horror stories we hear in our culture that depict nursing homes in a harsh and negative light, there are places in our communities that can provide activities, stimulation, compassion, and care that families cannot provide: hospice. Ideally, in these facilities we can pass away on our own terms, well cared for, comfortable, and surrounded by people we love. Finding these places and determining where you or a loved one might want to live is something all families should do before times get bad.

Several years ago as part of an NIH grant to explore medical decision making in dementia, I studied end-of-life care for persons with dementia. As part of the study, my co-author and I conducted interviews in hospice centers around the Cleveland area and asked family members with loved ones in hospice what suggestions they might make to others who would one day be in their position. Overwhelmingly, people emphasized that they wished they had known about and gotten involved in hospice much earlier, and that their physicians had educated them about the benefits of seeking hospice care. I would encourage you to seek out hospice facilities or at-home hospice programs in your area and get a feel for what your community offers. Additionally, many hospice facilities are in need of caring volunteers, and would warmly welcome your helping hand. If you are interested in volunteering for hospice but are unaware of any facilities in your area, visit the Web page of the Hospice Foundation of America at http://www.hospicefoundation.org/hospiceInfo/volunteer.asp.

Finally . . .

I have argued that coming to grips with our mortality can elevate the meaning in our lives. My next charge is for baby boomers to devote their later years to resisting two commonly held stereotypes about us: (1) that we are individualistic and selfish, and (2) that old age and retirement constitute an inevitable decline that brings about the cessation of work, increasing disability, deterioration of social networks, and a descent into oblivion. We can challenge both of these stereotypes by staying engaged in community and by giving ourselves to others—especially the generations that will follow us. Even if you are not at peak health, here are some outlets for your social contribution:

- Volunteer in your local school district.

- Lend a hand at your local food bank (recall that Ann Davidson's husband volunteered at a local food bank even as he was increasingly suffering from the symptoms of dementia).

- Offer your time at a free clinic.

- Serve as a mentor for a young person.

- Help coach a sports (Little League) team.

- Get a part-time job when you retire that will allow you to interact with others.

This list is not exhaustive. I can only exhort you to get involved in your community; what you elect to do is a matter of personal taste and availability. However you choose to invest your time and energy, let your actions invigorate not only you and your mind, but also your community.

> ## BOOMING NUMBERS OF VOLUNTEERS
>
> According to a recent study by researchers at Research Triangle Institute International, America's 77 million baby boomers have the highest volunteer participation rate of any demographic group. The study, funded by the Corporation for National and Community Service, was based on population surveys from 2002 to 2004 from the Bureau of Labor Statistics and the Census Bureau. Let's keep adding to those numbers!

PEAK 2: KEEPING YOUR HEAD IN THE CLOUDS: ENJOYING BEING A LIFELONG LEARNER

One of the most persistent themes in this book has been the importance of lifelong learning. Learning strengthens our cognitive reserve and saves us from intellectual stagnation. Increasingly, baby boomers are embracing their retirements as an opportunity for awakening and reinvention. More students in their forties, fifties, and beyond are enrolling in classes— seeking both career change and advancement, but also pursuing knowledge for personal enrichment. Understandably, many boomers may find the notion of being back on a college campus a bit harrowing. There are several programs that offer educational possibilities outside the ivory towers. OASIS (www.oasisnet.org) is a nonprofit that offers low-cost courses across the country to anyone fifty and over. Similarly, Elderhostel (www.elderhostel.org) is a program that enables aging persons to pursue learning opportunities in more than one hundred countries.

This knowledge can contribute to your personal edification, but it can also be applied to your community. An MBA or nonprofit management degree can be used to provide services in your community. Art or music skills that you develop can be used to help younger children cultivate lifelong skills and hobbies. A creative writing class may yield poems, stories, or books that can be of inspiration to other people.

PEAK 3: BUILDING A FIRM BASE THROUGH PREVENTION

Another strong theme in this book has been prevention. I have encouraged you to temper your hope about finding a "cure" for brain aging, and instead work toward the maintenance of your cognitive health throughout your life. My advice here is simple:

- Eat well.

- Exercise.

- Make sure your house is free of lead and other toxins.

- Work to improve the environmental health of your local and the global community.

- Expose your mind to challenging situations.

- Reduce stress.

- Maintain a strong sense of purpose.

- Protect your body and especially your head from injuries and accidents.

- Maintain your social networks.

But also remember that prevention means looking out for others. Addressing poverty and equity issues in your community is also part of prevention. Every individual mountain is part of a wider range. And every mountain range is rooted to the same earth.

The extension of prevention

A paper in the journal *Ageing Cell* showed that the lower your social standing, the faster you are likely to age. We need to concentrate our resources not only to prevent brain aging for ourselves, but also to help our poorest members give up smoking, lose weight, stay in school, and improve their diets, especially pregnant mothers and children whose brains are most vulnerable.

PEAK 4: ACTIVISM IN THE TWENTY-FIRST CENTURY

At their core, boomers still retain a spark of activism. Although this spark has dimmed since the 1960s as we have raised families and embarked on careers, baby boomers are sleeping giants whose reemergence as idealists in their retirement years can make a difference at all levels of our society. Issues of equity, equality, and environment will continue to be paramount to bettering mankind. There may always be senseless wars to oppose, politicians to keep in check, an environment to protect, and important causes to fight for. Move in the direction of your strongest beliefs, and remember that boomers are a potentially powerful voting bloc in many countries that will shape the contours of our collective future. If you need a further prod, studies have shown that engaging in politics and keeping apprised of world events may be protective against cognitive loss.

In the context of Alzheimer's disease, I would suggest that you encourage your local politicians to make life-span aging a priority issue on their agenda. I've already expressed my belief that money for brain aging should be more equitably distributed between the quest for the holy grail of "cure" and the search for our humanity in "care." I hope that after reading this book you now see the need for rethinking the use of our resources. Specifically, federal and state labor policies can help expand the pool of front-line caregivers. States must reach out to younger generations to increase the pool of committed workers and volunteers. We can create youth apprenticeship programs in nursing homes and assisted-living facilities in which high school students who wish to experience hands-on learning in the workplace in conjunction with classroom instruction are given the opportunity to have mentored on-the-job learning in an elder-care setting. Such programs can endow up-and-coming workers with the skills and competencies they will need to care for the growing number of elders in our society, and provide them with the knowledge, insight, and real-world experience they will need to take care of us in the future.

One of my patients had a son with whom I developed a strong working relationship. When it came time to put his mother in a nursing home, I gave him this advice: Make sure to form good initial relationships with the nursing home staff. They are humans just like anyone else, and the better relationship you form with them, the more inclined they will be to provide better care for your loved one. I also asked him to stay in contact with me even after his mother had been admitted to the nursing home, which had its own practicing physician. By maintaining a link between the primary physician and the nursing home physician you enable the two doctors to trade notes on your loved one. This communication can also result in your loved one receiving attention from the nursing home physician that she otherwise might not receive.

I would also urge you to e-mail the leaders of your local Alzheimer's disease chapter and express the belief that money raised for AD should be invested in care and prevention, and not just in the race for a cure that may never be forthcoming. To invest in caregiving means creating a compassionate infrastructure in our communities that can last for generations. Investing in prevention means more of us living longer with clearer minds. It also means protecting children and ensuring that they are given a good start in their development.

Beyond caregiving and prevention, we as a society need to reflect deeply on the communities of the future that will emerge to care for our elderly. New living arrangements—such as co-ops for the elderly, intergenerational living spaces, environmentally sound assisted-living facilities that promote cognitive stimulation and inclusion in community—must be at the forefront of our collective imaginations. I am not sure we want or can afford too much more institutional care for the frail elderly. If we can break down the barriers between those with dementing conditions and the healthy, and the young and other old, perhaps we can create living arrangements where people help each other across the cognitive and aging divides. Cooperative group arrangements supported by better architectural and environmental design may allow groups of mutually helping and helpful people to survive and thrive through cooperation arrangements. We are entering a challenging era as a human species. But humans are the most adaptable beings on the planet and I hope that we can rise to the challenges of the twenty-first century.

PEAK 5: EXPANDING INFORMATION TECHNOLOGY AMONG AGING INDIVIDUALS

The world is growing more and more dependent on information technology. Although it is a truism, if we fail to put in a modest effort to modernize, we will get left behind by the zeitgeist. So challenge yourself to stay abreast of technology, and to obtain at least the minimum amount of knowledge necessary to be computer-literate. The Internet is a truly amazing social phenomenon and will continue to enrich our lives if we continue to grow with it. Do not be left behind!

If you would like to seek out lessons on how to use the Internet, the community organizations for seniors will help you locate classes in your area. This is a worthy investment of your time. Besides the cognitive benefits conferred by searching for and taking in information, the Internet can be a common ground where we who are aging band together to redefine old age in the twenty-first century, not to mention change the story of Alzheimer's disease. When given basic, high-speed mobility on the Internet, patients and caregivers can find not only endless information at their fingertips but also a broad spectrum of stories told from the perspective of people who have dealt with what they themselves are going through. In the online communities that exist today, persons share techniques for handling doctor office visits, advice on choosing a doctor, and experience with medications and alternative treatments. Internet communities can create camaraderie, and counteract feelings of loneliness and despair that often affect aging individuals in our society, especially those who are widowed or who live separate from their families.

We have never before had the capacity to network with others that we do now, with billions of potential confidants a mere mouse click away. The Internet can be a great ally in bringing about a post-AD future: one in which aging individuals and their caregivers feel the continued empathy and presence of those who sympathize with the realities of aging and memory loss; one in which information about brain aging is readily available; one in which a multitude of stories about brain aging propagate in the place of the old stigmatizing and biologically reductionist myth of AD. We must challenge ourselves to learn how to navigate cyberspace.

TELL US YOUR STORY

We have launched a Web site, www.themythofalzheimers.com, and invite you to give it a visit, join our online community, and share your story with us. As my friend Harry Cayton has written, "If we can remember to acknowledge the complexity and multiplicity of the many narratives of dementia and the stories of individual lives which make them up we can diminish the tyranny of dementia."

The responsibility for modernizing along with technology is not just yours. I strongly urge the drug and health-care industry in general to enrich their business models by diversifying into the realm of information technology. Marketing products with clear consumer benefit will ultimately prove to be a more effective business plan than continuing to produce pills with only very modest benefit. Though a separate book could be written on potential products, I propose development in the following areas:

Computers as caregivers

Though it may initially conjure up images of the robot maid on *The Jetsons,* the notion of programming computers to offer caregiving assistance is not so far-fetched. Indeed, it behooves us to consider a future in which personal digital assistants (PDAs), computers, and smart houses can be refined and redesigned to be friendlier to persons with dementia in ways that address their personal needs, provide companionship, and protect their physical and mental frailty.

For instance, in most homes and in long-term-care facilities such as nursing homes, televisions are ubiquitous. If we replace televisions with interactive computer screens, a new world of therapeutic programming opens up. Instead of sitting idly as so often happens in assisted-living facilities, elderly persons could instead be engaged in what they are watching—actively "using" their minds instead of "losing" them passively. Interactive programming can usher in a new age of cognitively vital, person-centered care delivered in part by electronic technology.

Further, as is done in the nursing home in Oslo where Arne Naess lives, nursing homes of the future can use video cameras and GPS devices to track patients and monitor them if they get lost or fall. Personalized digital devices can hold individualized music, photo, and video files that can be used to stimulate or calm an individual with memory problems as the need arises. Integrating technology into our care for the elderly is an increasingly feasible endeavor. As a new generation of elderly boomers develop memory problems, they will already be more familiar with computers, and will appreciate the potential to enhance cognitive function and network with others.

Television network for the aging

Several years ago, Fox sent me the pilot episode for a new reality series they were developing called *Senior Moments*. Since most of the main characters—residents at a California retirement home—were former actors, the show was quite dramatic, with histrionic individuals involved in elaborate subplots that featured endless sniping and backstabbing and occasional tragedy. During the course of the pilot one of the residents was diagnosed with Alzheimer's disease, but his group of friends helped him resist the label.

Although to my knowledge the show never made it onto the air, its existence demonstrates that our broadcast companies are beginning to think differently about aging and its place in mainstream culture. Television is one of our country's most powerful means of mass communication. Currently we have television stations for everything under the sun: golf, classic sporting events, court proceedings, pop music, children, news, cooking, history, home repairs . . . Strange, then, how no channels have successful life-span aging as their theme.

It is obvious that television is a business, a private enterprise at work in a democratic society that is driven by mass-market demands, and even more obvious that advertisers are most interested in the coveted eighteen to forty-nine demographic because it is the major consumer group. But since the FCC licenses stations to operate in the "interest, convenience, and necessity"[2] of the community, it is quite puzzling that a channel devoted to successful aging (not to mention a show like *Senior Moments*) has yet to emerge.

If it is in fact economic pressures that dictate the content of our television stations, then it is not outlandish to think that the demographics of our rapidly aging country will create an impetus for programming that concentrates on what it means to grow old and to be old. Such a station could play a valuable role in people's lives, assisting them in coping with the challenges of old age and developing strategies for successful life-span aging. Polls show that people do not like to think of themselves as old, but as we continue to develop the concept that aging is a lifelong activity that is dynamic and full of the potential for self-transformation, such a channel would surely have broader appeal, and could help prompt wider cultural reflection on the aging, death, and dying process, and serve as a source of guidance and support for our aging elders. I challenge our broadcast networks to adapt their programming to reflect the aging baby boomer population and to serve a real public need.

THE FINAL PEAK

In this book, my co-author and I have stressed the importance of changing our minds about what we presently refer to as Alzheimer's disease. Our current myth limits our thoughts, actions, and behaviors, and fills our lives with unnecessary terror and angst. But the concept of aging is evolving, and with it our attitudes about growing older. Reframing Alzheimer's disease as brain aging and thus fundamentally altering the story we tell about cognitive loss can have profound effects on ourselves, our loved ones, our communities, our government policy, and our commerce. By placing ourselves on the continuum of brain aging and seeing it as a lifelong undertaking rather than an end-of-life "disease," we will find solidarity with all the vulnerable members in our society—from our children to our elders. This solidarity can provide an ethical impetus to protect our fellow human beings from the complex environmental and social factors that contribute to brain aging, while expanding our compassion for those in the later stages of senescence. By doing so, we will create a greater sense of responsibility for future generations and for our planet—a collective wisdom that will nurture our growth as a species.

Part of this responsibility will require us to think and act locally ("What can I do for my community and for myself?"), and more broadly ("How do all of our behaviors need to change on a larger scale?"). We must accept the limitations of science to cure brain aging and question the prudence of investing our resources in this quixotic pursuit. We must also question the excessive power that the pharmaceutical industry has over us and the tremendous waste that exists in our health-care systems and in our government, which spends billions of dollars on military campaigns and relatively little on the health of the public.

Through all these changes in our attitudes and behaviors, it must be remembered that suffering and death are inevitable. Our challenge is not to deny these aspects of our lives, but to think deeply about how we should prioritize our finite resources to the challenges we face. Thinking about the meaning of Alzheimer's disease is an exercise that may lead to greater wisdom. As we embrace the universality of cognitive aging and the inevitable decline in some abilities, we will come into contact with the deepest aspects of what it means to be human.

Baby boomers changed the world in the 1960s; now let's change the way we approach brain aging and care for aging persons—namely, everyone—as we grow older in the twenty-first century. I certainly wish us all well on our journey.

ACKNOWLEDGMENTS

We are first and foremost grateful to those human beings who rise above their own needs to care for others. As health practitioners and scholars committed to human health, we give our respect to those who celebrate the power of learning and apply the values of empathy and care, recognizing their contribution to quality of life.

To our teachers and collaborators in the scholarship journey, we express our thanks by including your ideas and influences in our lives and in this book. Recognizing that our message is not an uncontroversial one, we appreciate your willingness to allow us to develop these divergences in thought and action while in relationship with you. To those who resist our ideas, we acknowledge the importance of debate and discussion and your contributions to the conversation. To those who provided financial support for our careers and this project, we literally could not have done it without you. For those who actually contributed to the book by conducting research, editing our words, or providing us your images, we thank you. This book is a collaborative endeavor in the full depth of that word.

Peter would like to thank all his mentors through the years starting with his high school jobs at Johns Hopkins, continuing to Brown University, and then on to medical, doctoral, and postdoctoral work at Hopkins and in Boston—Charles Southwick's commitment to the environment and Jerry Frank's to healing the mind, in particular. To those for whom he has served as "boss," including those in the Alzheimer Center (now the University Memory and Aging Center) and Integrative Studies, he is grateful for their flexibility and tolerance of his energy level and travel schedule. Nationally, he has enjoyed many friendships among those who try to understand and help people with age-related dementias. He has also been fortunate to have many friends and collaborators in the international community. Prime among them are Martin Rossor and Akira Homma, who also arranged sabbaticals over the years. Sid Katz, a geriatrician and scholar of quality of life activity, and Van Rensselaer Potter, the inventor of bioethics, deserve special mention as wise elders. Oliver Sacks, Rachel Remen, and Rita Charon are inspiring examples of those who appreciate the power of narrative in its fullest extent. Cathy Greenblatt and Ed Kashi and Julie Winocur encouraged Peter's photographic eye. Anne Basting helped him move onto the stage more effectively. Rick Moody got his criticisms of science a bit more tempered while at the same time keeping him grounded in the sky. Gratitude is due to many younger scholars over the years and recently such folks as Jesse Ballenger, Jason Karlawish, Susie Sami, Danny George, Iahn Gonsenhauser, Heather Lindstrom, and others who allowed him occasional opportunities to offer advice to them as they developed their careers. He deeply appreciates the nurses and social workers who have guided him in trying to provide better care for elders at University Hospital Case Medical Center ElderHealth Center. Marian Patterson has offered steadfast neuropsychological and personal advice. Certain faculty members stand out in their consistent commitment to making the academic game enjoyable, notably Woody Gaines and Eric Junegst, who composed our sabbatical Limbo Café book planning (if not writing) group. Peter would also like to thank Stephen Post for the many ways he has taught him about the values of humility and altruism. A number of program coordinators, most recently Julia Rajcan, have provided able assistance and tolerated his active lifestyle. He also wishes to mention the dozens of graduate students in organizational behavior, and the younger learners in The Intergenerational School. You are both the energy and inspiration for wanting to change the world.

He would also like to thank his parents, Dennis and Joan Whitehouse, for their commitment to their family and to living life well. His father's interest in brain and behavior challenges in children inspired his own intellectual development, as did his mother's work with children as an educator and mother. His brothers and sisters, Michael, Heather, and Richard, have always been supportive of his life's work. His own children make working for a better future a pleasure and a necessity. Erin, a nurse, Meghan, a medical student, and Kirsten, a teacher, are walking good paths in life and contribute to his legacy. And, of course, the other in "our" is his wife, Cathy. As a fellow psychologist and educator she has been a colleague and collaborator. As one who is making a difference in the world through teaching urban city kids, she is his guiding light. Her love and support have made life possible, not to mention deeply worthwhile.

Daniel George would like to express the deepest of gratitude to his parents, Debra Rex and George George, and his sister, Emily George, for their ongoing support and encouragement (not to mention their attic), and would also like to express thanks to Sylvia Krinsky, Robert Molnar, and

Sarah Cofta for their editing help, as well as to Karen Bensing for her assistance in gathering library resources. Gratitude is also owed to his former professors at the College of Wooster, especially Dr. Thomas Tierney, his current professors at Oxford University, Elisabeth Hsu, Stanley Ulijaszek, and Sarah Harper, who have offered steady academic guidance, and to Peter Whitehouse, who is both mentor and friend. Thanks also to Andrew Porter, Darryl Wilkinson, Simon D'Alton, and Sarah Bennett for their friendship and sage words of advice and encouragement over Warnock meals and cups of tea, to the fivefifteen fellows for their support and constant comic relief, to Frauke Fechner and Anna-Lena Scholz for their help with German pronunciation, and to all our friends and colleagues in Integrative Studies who have been so supportive.

And last, we would both like to thank our agent, Gail Ross, and her colleague Howard Yoon for introducing us to the world of book publishing, and to Sheila Curry Oakes and Diane Reverand at St. Martin's Press for their commitment to our idea and their wise editing advice.

Appendix

Suggested Readings

Angell, Marcia. *The Truth About the Drug Companies: How They Deceive Us and What to Do About It.*

Basting, Anne. *Forget Memory.*

Bellenger, Jessie. *Do We Have a Pill for That?*

———. *Self, Senility and Alzheimer's Disease in Modern America: A History.*

Bond, J., Cormer, L. *Quality of Life and Older People.*

Charon, Rita. *Stories Matter: The Role of Narrative in Medical Ethics.*

Cohen, Gene. *The Creative Age: Awakening Human Potential in the Second Half of Life.*

———. *The Mature Mind: The Positive Power of the Aging Brain.*

Davidson, Ann. *Alzheimer's: A Love Story.*

———. *A Curious Kind of Widow.*

Fuchs, Elinor. *Making an Exit: A Mother-Daughter Drama with Alzheimer's, Machine Tools, and Laughter.*

Harding, N. H., Palfrey, C. *The Social Construction of Dementia: Confused Professionals.*

Hollis, James. *Finding Meaning in the Second Half of Life.*

Kassirer, J. *On the Take: How Medicine's Complicity with Big Business Can Endanger Your Health.*

Kitwood, Tom. *Dementia Reconsidered: The Person Comes First.*

Levine, Judith. *Do You Remember Me? A Father, a Daughter, and a Search for the Self.*

Potter, V. R. *Bioethics Bridge to the Future.*

———. *Global Bioethics.*

Remen, R. *Kitchen Table Wisdom: Stories That Heal.*

Sabat, S. *The Experience of AD: Life Through a Tangled Veil.*

Sacks, Oliver. *The Man Who Mistook His Wife for a Hat: And Other Clinical Tales.*

Turner, Mark. *The Literary Mind: The Origins of Thought and Language.*

Whitehouse, P. J., et al. *Concepts of Alzheimer's Disease: Biological, Clinical and Cultural Perspectives.*

Wykle, M., Whitehouse, P., Morris, D. L. *Successful Aging Through the Lifespan: Intergenerational Issues in Health.*

Resources: Organizations (Courtesy of the National Institute on Aging)

Alzheimer's Association. The Alzheimer's Association is a national nonprofit organization with a network of local chapters that provide education and support for people diagnosed with AD, their families, and caregivers. Chapters offer referrals to local resources and services, and sponsor support groups and educational programs. Online and print publications are also available.

> Alzheimer's Association
> 225 North Michigan Avenue, Suite 1700
> Chicago, IL 60601
> Web site: www.alz.org

Alzheimer's Disease Cooperative Study. The Alzheimer's Disease Cooperative Study (ADCS) is the result of a cooperative agreement between the National Institute on Aging (NIA) and the University of California, San Diego, to advance research in the development of drugs to treat AD. The ADCS is a consortium of medical research centers and clinics working to develop clinical trials of medicines to treat behavioral symptoms of AD, improve cognition, slow the rate of decline of AD, delay the onset of AD, or prevent the disease altogether. The ADCS also develops new and more reliable ways to evaluate patients enrolled in clinical trials.

> Alzheimer's Disease Cooperative Study
> University of California, San Diego
> 9500 Gilman Drive
> La Jolla, CA 92093-0949
> 858-622-5880
> Web site: http://adcs.ucsd.edu

Alzheimer's Disease Education and Referral (ADEAR) Center. The ADEAR Center, part of the NIA, provides publications and information on AD, including booklets on caregiving, fact sheets and reports on research findings, a database of clinical trials, recommended reading lists, and the Progress Report on Alzheimer's Disease. Information specialists provide referrals to local AD resources.

> Alzheimer's Disease Education and Referral (ADEAR) Center
> PO Box 8250

Silver Spring, MD 20907
1-800-438-4380
Web site: www.nia.nih.gov/alzheimers

Children of Aging Parents. Children of Aging Parents is a nonprofit organization that provides information and referrals for nursing homes, retirement communities, elder-law attorneys, adult-day-care centers, medical insurance providers, respite care, assisted-living centers, and state and county agencies. Also offered are fact sheets on various topics, a bimonthly newsletter, conferences and workshops, support group referrals, and a speaker's bureau.

Children of Aging Parents
1609 Woodbourne Road, Suite 302A
Levittown, PA 19057-1511
1-800-227-7294
Web site: www.caps4caregivers.org

Eldercare Locator. The Eldercare Locator is a nationwide directory assistance service helping older people and their caregivers locate local support and resources. It is funded by the U.S. Administration on Aging, whose Web site at www.aoa.gov also features AD information for families, caregivers, and health professionals.

Eldercare Locator
1-800-677-1116
Web site: www.eldercare.gov

Family Caregiver Alliance. The Family Caregiver Alliance (FCA) is a nonprofit organization that offers support services for those caring for adults with AD, stroke, traumatic brain injuries, and other cognitive disorders. FCA programs and services include an Information Clearinghouse for FCA's publications.

Family Caregiver Alliance
690 Market Street, Suite 600
San Francisco, CA 94104
415-434-3388
Web site: www.caregiver.org

National Hospice and Palliative Care Organization (NHPCO). NHCPO is a nonprofit membership organization working to enhance the quality of life for individuals who are terminally ill and advocating for people in the final stage of life. Contact NHPCO for information, resources, and referrals to local hospice services. Publications, fact sheets, and Web site resources are available on many topics, including how to find and evaluate hospice services.

> National Hospice and Palliative Care Organization
> 1700 Diagonal Road, Suite 625
> Alexandria , VA 22314
> 1-800-658-8898 (toll-free help line)
> Web site: www.nhpco.org

National Institute on Aging (NIA). Part of the National Institutes of Health (NIH), the NIA is the federal government's lead agency for research on AD. NIA also offers information about health and aging, including the Age Page series and the NIA Exercise Kit, which contains an eighty-page exercise guide and forty-eight-minute closed-captioned video. Caregivers can find many Age Pages on the Web site.

> National Institute on Aging Information Center
> PO Box 8057
> Gaithersburg, MD 20898-8057
> 1-800-222-2225
> 1-800-222-4225 (TTY)
> Web site: www.nia.nih.gov

National Library of Medicine. Part of NIH, the National Library of Medicine is the world's largest medical library with six million items, including books, journals, technical reports, manuscripts, microfilms, photographs, and images. A large searchable health information database of biomedical journals, called MEDLINE/PubMed, is accessible via the Internet. A service called MEDLINEplus links the public to general information about AD and caregiving, plus many other sources of consumer health information, including a searchable clinical trials database located at http://clinicaltrials.gov.

> National Library of Medicine
> 8600 Rockville Pike
> Bethesda, MD 20894

1-888-346-3656
Web site: www.nlm.nih.gov

Well Spouse Foundation. Well Spouse Foundation is a nonprofit organization that gives support to spouses and partners of the chronically ill and/or disabled. Well Spouse maintains support groups, publishes a bimonthly newsletter, and helps organize letter-writing programs to help members deal with the effects of isolation.

Well Spouse Foundation
63 West Main Street, Suite H
Freehold, NJ 07728
1-800-838-0879
Web site: www.wellspouse.org

Notes

Preface

1. Turner, M. *The Literary Mind*. Oxford: Oxford University Press, 1996, p. 5.
2. Ferri, C. P., et al. 2005. "Global Prevalence of Dementia: A Delphi Consensus Study." *Lancet* 366(9503):2112–17.
3. There is a popular literature in the Alzheimer's field which argues that persons with AD digress in fairly predictable "stages." See Reisberg, B., et al., 1984, "Functional Staging of Dementia of the Alzheimer Type," *Annals of the New York Academy of Sciences* 435:481–83, and Reisberg, B., et al. 1989, "The Stage Specific Temporal Course of Alzheimer's Disease: Functional and Behavioral Concomitants Based upon Cross-Sectional and Longitudinal Observation," in Iqbal, K., Wisniewski, H. M., Winblad, B., eds., *Alzheimer's Disease and Related Disorders* (New York: Liss), pp. 23–41.
4. Caplan, A., McCartney, J., Sisti, D. *Health, Disease, and Illness: Concepts in Medicine*. Washington, D.C.: Georgetown University Press, 2004, Chapter 4.

Introduction: Revealing the Myth of Alzheimer's

1. Lévi-Strauss, C. *Myth and Meaning: Cracking the Code of Culture*. New York: Schocken Books, 1978.
2. Kitwood, T. *Dementia Reconsidered: The Person Comes First*. Philadelphia: Open University Press, 1997, p. 118.
3. Fulford, R. *The Triumph of Narrative: Storytelling in the Age of Mass Culture*. Toronto: Anansi, 1999.
4. Annas, G. 1995. "Reframing the Debate on Health Care Reform by Replacing Our Metaphors." *New England Journal of Medicine* 332:745–48.
5. Bahro, M., et al. 1995. "How Do Patients with Alzheimer's Disease Cope with Their Illness? A Clinical Experience Report." *Journal of the American Geriatrics Society* 43(1):41–46.
6. Martin, E. *The Woman in the Body*. Boston: Beacon, 1987, p. 203.

Chapter 1: A Gateway to the Future of Old Age

1. Sabat, S. R. 2002. "Epistemological Issues in the Study of Insight in People with Alzheimer's Disease." *Dementia* 1(11):279–93.

2. Kitwood, T. *Dementia Reconsidered: The Person Comes First.* Philadelphia: Open University Press, 1997.

3. Kolata, G. 2006. "Old but Not Frail: A Matter of Heart and Head." *New York Times*, October 5, section A.

4. Kitwood, op. cit., p. 3.

5. Gollaher, D. L. 1994. "From Ritual to Science: The Medical Transformation of Circumcision in America." *Journal of Social History* 28(1):5–36.

6. Kitwood, op. cit., p. 141.

7. Katzman, R., Bick, K. *Alzheimer Disease: The Changing View.* San Diego: Academic Press, 2000, p. 195. Fox, P. J. 1986. "Alzheimer's Disease: An Historical Overview." *American Journal of Alzheimer's Care*, Fall, p. 18.

8. Franzen, J. "My Father's Brain." *The New Yorker*, September 10, 2001, p. 85.

9. Davidson, A. *A Curious Kind of Widow.* McKinleyville, CA: Daniel & Daniel Publishers, 2006, p. 19.

10. Griffin, J., Fuhrer, R., Stansfeld, S. A., Marmot, M. G. 2002. "The Importance of Low Control at Work and Home on Depression and Anxiety: Do These Effects Vary by Gender and Social Class?" *Social Science and Medicine* 54(5):783–98.

11. Midgley, M. *Science and Poetry.* London: Routledge, 2001, p. 120.

12. Alzheimer's Association, http://www.alz.org/AboutAD/statistics.asp (accessed October 12, 2006).

13. Ibid.

14. Valliant, G., Mukamal, K. 2001. "Successful Aging." *American Journal of Psychiatry* 158(6): 839.

15. Ferri, C. P., et al. 2005. "Global Prevalence of Dementia: A Delphi Consensus Study." *Lancet* 366(9503):2112–17.

16. Rattan, S. 2005. "Anti-Aging Strategies: Prevention or Therapy?" *Science and Society,* EMBO reports, vol. 6, p. S25.

17. Cayton, H. 2004. "Telling Stories: Choices and Challenges on the Journey of Dementia." *Dementia* 3(1):9–17.

18. MacIntyre, A. *After Virtue: A Study in Moral Theory.* South Bend, Ind.: University of Notre Dame Press, 1981.

19. Goffman, E. *Stigma: Notes on the Management of Spoiled Identity.* New York: Prentice Hall, 1963.

20. Waxler, N. E. 1979. "Is Outcome for Schizophrenia Better in Nonindustrial Societies? The Case of Sri Lanka." *Journal of Nervous and Mental Disease* 167(3):144–58.

Chapter 2: Alzheimer's 101: Taming the Scientific Story of AD

1. Cayton, H. 2004. "Telling Stories: Choices and Challenges on the Journey of Dementia." *Dementia* 3(1).

2. Winter, R. "Fictional-Critical Criting." In Nias, J., Groundwater-Smoth, S., eds., *The Enquiring Teacher.* London: Falmer, 1988, pp. 231–48.

3. Maguire, E. A., et al. 2000. "Navigation-Related Structural Change in the

Hippocampi of Taxi Drivers." *Proceedings of the National Academy of Sciences of the United States of America* 97(8):4398–4403.

4. *Alzheimer's Disease: Unraveling the Mystery*. December 2003. National Institute on Aging, U.S. Department of Health and Human Services, No. 02–3782.

5. Lee, H. G. 2006. "Amyloid Beta: The Alternate Hypothesis." *Current Alzheimer's Research* 3(1):75–80. Rottkamp, C. A., et al. 2002. "The State Versus Amyloid-Beta: The Trial of the Most Wanted Criminal in Alzheimer Disease." *Peptides* 23(7):1333–41. Koudinov, A. R., Berezov, T. T. "Alzheimer's Amyloid-Beta Is an Essential Synaptic Protein, Not Neurotoxic Junk." *Acta Neurobiological Experimentalis* 64:71–79.

6. Lee, H. G., et al. 2004. "Challenging the Amyloid Cascade Hypothesis: Senile Plaques and Amyloid-ß as Protective Adaptations to Alzheimer Disease." *Annals of the New York Academy of Sciences* 1019:1–4.

7. Smith, M. A., et al. May 25, 2002. "Predicting the Failure of Amyloid-Beta Vaccine." *Lancet* 359(9320):1864–65.

8. Knopman, D. S., et al. 2004. "Neuropathology of Cognitively Normal Elderly." *Journal of Neuropathology and Experimental Neurology* 62:1087–95.

9. Stein, M. *This Room Is Yours*. New York: Permanent Press, 2004, pp. 75–76.

10. Peterson, R., et al. 2005. "Vitamin E and Donepezil for the Treatment of Mild Cognitive Impairment." *New England Journal of Medicine* 352:2379–88.

11. Miller, E. R., III, et al. 2005. "Meta-Analysis: High-Dosage Vitamin E Supplementation May Increase All-Cause Mortality." *Annals of Internal Medicine* 142:37–46.

12. Singh, V. K., Guthikinda, P. 1997. "Circulating Cytokines in AD." *Journal of Psychiatry* 31(6):657–60. Weaver, J. D., et al. 2002. "Interleukin-6 and Risk of Cognitive Decline: MacArthur Studies of Successful Aging." *Neurology* 59(3):371–78.

13. Mayeaux, R., et al. 1995. "Synergistic Effects of Traumatic Head Injury and Apolipoprotein-E4 in Patients with Alzheimer's Disease." *Neurology* 45:555–57.

14. Esiri, M., Nagy, Z. "Neuropathology." In Jacoby, R., Oppenheimer, C., eds., *Psychiatry in the Elderly*, 3rd ed. Oxford: Oxford University Press, 2002, pp. 102–24.

Chapter 3: The Troubling Legacy of Dr. Alois Alzheimer and Auguste D.

1. Leroux, C. July 22, 1997. "The Case of Auguste D." *Chicago Tribune*, p. E1.

2. Maurer, K., Volk, S., Gerbaldo, H. 1997. "Auguste D. and Alzheimer's Disease." *Lancet* 349:1546–49.

3. Maurer, K., Maurer, U. *Alzheimer: The Life of a Physician and the Career of a Disease*. New York: Columbia University Press, 2003, pp. 53–54.

4. Ibid., p. 19.

5. Perusini, G. "Uber Klinisch und Histologisch Eigenartige Psychische Erkrankungen des Späteren Lebensalters." In Nissl, F., Alzheimer, A., eds., *Histologische und Histopathologische Arbeiten*. Jena: Verlag Fischer, 1909, pp. 297–351.

6. Maurer and Maurer, op. cit., pp. 115–16.

7. Ibid., p. 170.

8. Ibid., p. 169.

9. Kraepelin, E. *Psychiatric: Ein Lehrbuch für Studierende und Artze*. Barth, Leipzig, 1910.

10. Maurer and Maurer, op. cit., p. 281.

11. Whitehouse, P. J., et al. *Concepts of Alzheimer's Disease: Biological, Clinical and Cultural Perspectives*. Baltimore: Johns Hopkins University Press, 2000, p. 41.

12. Kuhn, T. S. *The Structure of Scientific Revolutions*. Chicago: University of Chicago Press, 1962, p. 75.

13. Berrios, G. E. 1990. "Alzheimer's Disease: A Conceptual History." *International Journal of Geriatric Psychiatry* 5(6):355–65.

14. Schorer, C. E. 1985. "Historical Essay: Kraepelin's Description of Alzheimer's Disease." *International Journal of Aging and Human Development* 21(3):238.

15. Berrios, G. E. 1990. "Alzheimer's Disease: A Conceptual History." *International Journal of Geriatric Psychiatry* 5(6):355–65.

16. Maurer and Maurer, op. cit., pp. 165, 218.

17. Gay, P. *Freud: A Life for Our Time*. London: Little Books, 2006, p. 85.

18. Thomas, M., Isaac, M. 1987. "Alois Alzheimer: A Memoir." *Trends in Neurosciences* 10(8).

19. Kuhn, op. cit., p. 136.

Chapter 4: The Birth of the Alzheimer's Empire

1. Ballenger, J. *Self, Senility, and Alzheimer's Disease in Modern America: A History*. Baltimore: Johns Hopkins University Press, 2006, p. 68

2. Ibid.

3. Ibid., p. 49.

4. U.S. Bureau of the Census. *Statistical Abstract of the United States: 1970*, 91st ed. Washington, D.C.: U.S. Government Printing Office, 1970.

5. Ballenger, op. cit., p. 446.

6. Fox, P. 1989. "Rise of the Alzheimer's Disease Movement." *Milbank Quarterly* 67(1):82.

7. Ballenger, J. "The Stigmatization of Old Age in the US." In *Thinking About Dementia: Culture, Loss and the Anthropology of Senility*. New Brunswick, N.J.: Rutgers University Press, 2006.

8. Fox, op. cit., p. 89.

9. Ballenger, op. cit.

10. Ibid., p. 193.

11. Nichter, M. December 1981. "Idioms of Distress: Alternatives in the Expression of Psychosocial Distress: A Case Study from South India." *Culture, Medicine and Psychiatry* 5(4):379–408.

12. Concepts 220.

13. Yahoo! press release: "Sargent and Mark Shriver to Present the First-Ever Eunice and Sargent Shriver 'Profile in Dignity Award,'" March 23, 2004.

14. www.alz.org.

15. www.alz.org/national/documents/safereturn-lawenforcement.pdf.

16. "Your Health in the 21st Century." *Newsweek*, June 20, 2005.

17. Khachaturian, Z. *Alzheimer's Disease: Cause(s), Diagnosis, Treatment, and Care.* New York: CRC-Taylor & Francis, 1996.

18. Khachaturian, Z. 1997. "Plundered Memories." *The Sciences* 37(4):21–25.

19. Kitwood, T. *Dementia Reconsidered.* Philadelphia: Open University Press, 1997, pp. 5–6.

20. Ibid., p. 69.

21. Story paraphrased from Golub, E., *The Limits of Medicine: How Science Shapes Our Hope for the Cure.* Chicago: University of Chicago Press, 1994.

22. Kitwood, op. cit., p. 36.

Chapter 5: Waiting for Godot: Alzheimer's Treatments Past and Present

1. Lock, M., Lloyd, S., Prest, J. "Genetics and Alzheimer's Research." In *Thinking About Dementia: Culture, Loss and the Anthropology of Senility.* New Brunswick, N.J.: Rutgers University Press, 2006, p. 129.

2. Alzheimer's Association: Fact Sheet 2006, p. 1.

3. "Eisai Reports Results from Latest Donepezil Study in Vascular Dementia." Press release No. 06–10, March 16, 2006, http://www.eisai.co.jp/enews/enews200609 .html (accessed December 19, 2006). "Galantamine (Reminyl)-Possible Increased Mortality in Patients with Mild Cognitive Impairment." University of Utah Health Care Hospitals and Clinics Drug Information Service report for April 5, 2005, http://uuhsc.utah.edu/pharmacy/alerts/81.html (accessed December 19, 2006).

4. Yesavage, J. A., et al. 2002. "Donepezil and Flight Simulator Performance: Effects on Retention of Complex Skills." *Neurology* 59(1):123–25.

5. Hofman, A. J. C., et al. 1998. "Smoking and Risk of Dementia and Alzheimer's Disease in a Population-Based Cohort Study: The Rotterdam Study." *Lancet* 351(9119):1840.

6. Logsdon, R. G., et al. 2002. "Assessing Quality of Life in Older Adults with Cognitive Impairment." *Psychosomatic Medicine* 64(3):510–19. Teri, L., et al. 2003. "Exercise Plus Behavior Management in Patients with Alzheimer's Disease: A Controlled Clinical Trial." *JAMA* 290(15):2015–22.

7. U.S. Department of Health and Human Services, Public Health Service, National Institutes of Health, National Institute on Aging. *Genes, Lifestyles and Crossword Puzzles: Can Alzheimer's Disease Be Prevented?* May 2005, NIH Publication No. 05-5503.

8. Jobst, K. A., Shostak, D., Whitehouse, P. J. 1999. "Diseases of Meaning: Manifestations of Health, and Metaphor." *The Journal of Alternative and Complementary Medicine* 5:6:495–502.

9. Durga, J., et al. January 20, 2007. "Effect of 3-Year Folic Acid Supplementation on Cognitive Function in Older Adults in the FACIT Trial: A Randomised, Double Blind, Controlled Trial." *Lancet* 369(9557):208–16.

10. Abramson, J. *Overdosed America: The Broken Promise of American Medicine.* New York: HarperCollins, 2004.

Chapter 6: A Brave New World of Genetics and Molecular Medicine?

1. "President Clinton Announces the Completion of the First Survey of the Entire Human Genome: Hails Public and Private Efforts Leading to This Historic Achievement." White House press release, June 25, 2000.

2. Cupples, L. A., et al. 2004. "Estimating Risk Curves for First-Degree Relatives of Patients with Alzheimer's Disease: The REVEAL Study." *Genetic Medicine* 6(4):192–96. Roberts, J. S., et al. 2005. "Genetic Risk Assessment for Adult Children of People with Alzheimer's Disease: The Risk Evaluation and Education for Alzheimer's Disease (REVEAL) Study." *Journal of Geriatric Psychiatry and Neurology* 18:250–55.

3. Lock, M., et al. "Genetics and Alzheimer Research." In A. Leibing and L. Cohen, eds., *Thinking About Dementia: Culture, Loss and the Anthropology of Senility.* New Brunswick, N.J.: Rutgers University Press, 2006, p. 132.

4. "Genetic Susceptibility and Alzheimer's Disease: The Penetrance and Uptake of Genetic Knowledge." In A. Leibling snd L. Cohen, eds., op. cit., pp.123–55.

5. Katz, D. 2006. "Taking Vitamins Based on Race: GenSpec Introduces Race-Specific Vitamins." ABC news online, April 12, 2006, http://abcnews.go.com/GMA/Health/story?id=1834160 (accessed April 14, 2006).

6. Morris, J. April–June 2005. "Dementia Update 2005." *Alzheimer's Disease and Associated Disorders* 19(2):100–117.

7. Angell, M. *The Truth About the Drug Companies.* New York: Random House, 2004, p. 20.

8. Cha, S. August 1, 2005. "Doctors Must Say 'No': Accepting Gifts from Pharmaceutical Firms Muddies Judgment, Violates Patients' Trust." Syndicated article printed in *Cleveland Plain Dealer,* Section B.

9. Whitehouse, P. J. 2003. "The Rebirth of Bioethics: Extending the Original Formulations of Van Rensselaer Potter." *American J Bioethics* 3(4):W26–W31.

Chapter 7: Identifying Who Needs a Prescription for Memory Loss

1. Traphagan, J. "Being a Good Rojin." In *Thinking About Dementia: Culture, Loss and the Anthropology of Senility.* New Brunswick, N.J.: Rutgers University Press, 2006, p. 274.

2. Reprinted with permission from www.alz.org.

3. Mayberg, H. S., et al. "Neuropsychiatric Aspects of Mood and Affective Disorders." In *Neuropsychiatry and Clinical Neurosciences.* Washington, D.C.: American Psychiatric Publishing Inc., 2002, pp. 1021–48.

4. Rapp, M. A., et al. 2006. "Increased Hippocampal Plaques and Tangles in Patients with Alzheimer's Disease with a Lifetime History of Major Depression." *Archives of General Psychiatry* 63:161–67.

5. Troller, J., Valenzuela, M. 2001. "Brain Ageing in the New Millennium." *Australian and New Zealand Journal of Psychiatry* 35:788–805.

6. According to this theory, a decrease in mitochondrial processing can promote mitochondrial mutations. It is theorized that this can accelerate the production of reactive oxygen species, i.e., free radicals.

7. Kleim, J. A., et al. January 15, 1997. "Learning-Dependent Synaptic Modifications in the Cerebellar Cortex of the Adult Rat Persist for at Least Four Weeks." *Journal of Neuroscience* 17(2):717–21.

8. Li, S. C. 2003. "Biocultural Orchestration of Developmental Plasticity Across Levels: The Interplay of Biology and Culture in Shaping the Mind and Behavior Across the Life Span." *Psychological Bulletin* 129(2):171–94.

Chapter 8: Preparing for a Doctor's Visit

1. Basting, A. D. 2003. "Looking Back from Loss: Views of the Self in Alzheimer's Disease." *Journal of Aging Studies* 17(1):87–99.

2. Sternberg, R. J., Jordan, J. *A Handbook of Wisdom: Psychological Perspectives.* Cambridge: Cambridge University Press, 2005.

3. Quoted in Clare L., 2003. "Managing Threats to Self: Awareness in Early Stage Alzheimer's Disease," *Social Science and Medicine* 57:1017–29.

Chapter 9: A Prescription for Successful Aging Across Your Life Span

1. Berrino, F. May–June 2002. "Western Diet and Alzheimer's Disease." *Epidemiology Prevention* 26(3):107–15.

2. Grant, W. B. November 1999. "Dietary Links to Alzheimer's Disease." *Alzheimer's Disease Review* 1(4–5):197–201.

3. O'Keefe, J. R., Cordain, L. 2004. "Cardiovascular Disease Resulting from a Diet and Lifestyle at Odds with Our Paleolithic Genome: How to Become a 21st Century Hunter-Gatherer." *Mayo Clinic Proceedings* 79(7):101–8.

4. Eaton, S. B., Eaton, S. B., III. "Hunter-Gatherers and Human Health." In *The Cambridge Encyclopedia of Hunters and Gatherers.* Cambridge: Cambridge University Press, 1999, p. 449.

5. McMichael, A. J. *Human Frontiers, Environments, and Disease.* Cambridge: Cambridge University Press, 2001.

6. Schaefer, E. J., et al. 2006. "Plasma Phosphatidylcholine Docosahexaenoic Acid Content and Risk of Dementia and Alzheimer Disease: The Framingham Heart Study." *Archives of Neurology* 63:1545–50.

7. Morris, M. C., et al. 2005. "Fish Consumption and Cognitive Decline with Age in a Large Community Study." *Archives of Neurology* 62.12.noc50161.

8. Morris, M. C., et al. 2004. "Dietary Fat Intake and 6-Year Cognitive Change in an Older Biracial Community Population." *Neurology* 62:1573–79.

9. Simopoulos, A. P. 1999. "Evolutionary Aspects of Omega-3 Fatty Acids in the Food Supply." *Prostaglandins, Leukotrienes and Essential Fatty Acids* 60(5–6):421–29. Morris, J. April–June 2005. "Dementia Update 2005." *Alzheimer's Disease and Associated Disorders* 19(2).

10. De Caterina, R., Basta, G. 2001. "N-3 Fatty Acids and the Inflammatory Response—Biological Background." *European Heart Journal Supplement* 3 (Supplement D):D42–D49. Hann M., Wallace, R. 2004. "Can Dementia Be Prevented? Brain Aging in a Population-Based Context." *Annual Review of Public Health* 25:1–24. Simopoulos, op. cit., pp. 421–29.

11. Mozaffarian, D. 2006. "Fish Intake, Contaminants, and Human Health." *JAMA* 296(15):1885–99.

12. EPA dietary advice on fish, http://www.epa.gov/waterscience/fishadvice/advice.html.

13. Ruitenberg, A., et al. 2002. "Alcohol Consumption and Risk of Dementia: The Rotterdam Study." *Lancet* 359(9303):281–86.

14. Scarmeas, N., et al. 2006. "Mediterranean Diet and Risk for Alzheimer's Disease." *American Neurological Association* 59(6):912–21.

15. Morris, M. C., et al. 2006. "Associations of Vegetable and Fruit Consumption with Age-Related Cognitive Change." *Neurology* 67(8):1370–76.

16. Ganguli, M., et al. 2000. "Apolipoprotein E Polymorphism and Alzheimer's Disease: The Indo-US Cross-National Dementia Study." *Archives of Neurology* 57:824–30.

17. Tze-Pin Ng, et al. 2006. "Curry Consumption and Cognitive Function in the Elderly." *American Journal of Epidemiology* 164(9):898–906.

18. Zhu, H., Guo, Q., Mattson, M. P. 1999. "Dietary Restriction Protects Hippocampal Neurons Against the Death-Promoting Action of Presenilin-1 Mutation." *Brain Res* 842(1):224–29.

19. Pasinetti, G. M., et al. 2007. "Caloric Intake and Alzheimer's Disease: Experimental Approaches and Therapeutic Implications." *Interdisciplinary Topics in Gerontology* 35:159–75.

20. Waterland, R., Garza, C. 1999. "Potential Mechanisms of Metabolic Imprinting That Lead to Chronic Disease." *American Journal of Clinical Nutrition* 69(2):179–97.

21. Horwood, J. L., Fergusson, D. M. 1998. "Breastfeeding and Later Cognitive and Academic Outcomes." *Pediatrics* 101(1):e9.

22. Rodgers, B. 1978. "Feeding in Infancy and Later Ability and Attainment: A Longitudinal Study." *Journal of Developmental Medicine and Child Neurology* 20:421–26.

23. Uauy, R., De Andraca, I. 1995. "Human Milk and Breast Feeding for Optimal Mental Development." *British Journal of Nutrition* 125:2278S–80S.

24. Uauy, R., Peirano, P. 1999. "Breast Is Best: Human Milk Is the Optimal Food for Brain Development." *American Journal of Clinical Nutrition* 70:433–34.

25. O'Keefe and Cordain, op. cit., pp. 101–8.

26. Trejo, J. L., Carro, E., Torres-Alemán, I. March 1, 2001. "Circulating Insulin-Like Growth Factor I Mediates Exercise-Induced Increases in the Number of New Neurons in the Adult Hippocampus." *Journal of Neuroscience* 21(5):1628–34.

27. Tinetti, M. E., et al. September 29, 1994. "A Multifactorial Intervention to Reduce the Risk of Falling Among Elderly People Living in the Community." *New England Journal of Medicine* 331(13):821–27. Stuck, A. E., et al. 1999. "Risk Factors for Functional Status Decline in Community-Living Elderly People: A Systematic Literature Review." *Social Science and Medicine* 48(4):445–69. Appel, L. J., et al. Writing Group for the PREMIER Collaborative Research Group. 2003. "Effects of Comprehensive Lifestyle Modification on Blood Pressure Control: Main Results of the PREMIER Clinical Trial." *JAMA* 289(16):2083–93. Kramer, A. F., et al. 2005. "Fitness, Aging and Neurocognitive Function." *Neurobiology of Aging* 26:S124–27.

28. Peeke, P. *Body for Life for Women.* New York: Rodale, 2005.

29. Larson, E. B., et al. January 17, 2006. "Exercise in People Age 65 Years and Older Is Associated with Lower Risk for Dementia." *Annals of Internal Medicine* 144(2):73–81.

30. Barker, D. "The Origins of Coronary Heart Disease in Early Life." In Henry, C. J. K., Ulijaszek, S., eds., *Long Term Consequences of Early Enviroment: Growth, Development and the Lifespan Developmental Perspective.* Cambridge: Cambridge University Press, 1996.

31. Grandjean, P., Landrigan, P. J. December 16, 2006. "Developmental Neurotoxicity of Industrial Chemicals." *Lancet* 368(9553):2167.

32. Barthes, D., et al., eds. 1973. *Proceedings of International Symposium. Environmental Health Aspects of Lead.* Commission of European Community, Luxembourg, pp. 1, 168.

33. Nriagu, J. O., ed. *The Biogeochemistry of Lead in the Environment. Part A. Ecological Cycles.* Amsterdam: Elsevier/North Holland Biomedical Press, 1978, p. 422. De Michele, S. J. 1984. "Nutrition of Lead." *Comparative Biochemistry and Physiology* 78A:401–8.

34. Basha, M. R., et al. January 26, 2005. "The Fetal Basis of Amyloidogenesis: Exposure to Lead and Latent Overexpression of Amyloid Precursor Protein and Beta-Amyloid in the Aging Brain." *Journal of Neuroscience* 25(4):823–29.

35. Needleman, H. L., et al. 2002. "Bone Lead Levels in Adjudicated Delinquents. A Case Control Study." *Neurotoxicology and Teratology* 24:711–17.

36. Lamphear, B. P., et al. 2005. "Low-Level Environmental Lead Exposure and Children's Intellectual Function: An International Pooled Analysis." *Environmental Health Perspectives* 13:894–99.

37. Greater Cleveland Lead Advisory Board, 2006, http://www.clevelandhealth.org/activeserverpages/environment/leadelimination.asp (accessed December 15, 2006).

38. Grandjean and Landrigan, op. cit., pp. 167–78.

39. National Research Council. *Toxicological Effects of Methylmercury.* Washington, D.C.: National Academy Press, 2000.

40. Landrigan, P. J. 1981. "Arsenic—State of the Art." *American Journal of Industrial Medicine* 2:5–14.

41. Grandjean and Landrigan, op. cit., p. 2172.

42. Ibid., p. 2173.

43. Rohlman, D. S., et al. 2005. "Neurobehavioral Performance in Preschool Children from Agricultural and Non-Agricultural Communities in Oregon and North Carolina." *Neurotoxicology* 26(6):589–98.

44. Guillette, E. A., et al. 1998. "An Anthropological Approach to the Evaluation of Preschool Children Exposed to Pesticides in Mexico." *Environmental Health Perspectives* 106:347–53.

45. Barlow, et al. 2007. "The Gestational Environment and Parkinson's Disease: Evidence for Neurodevelopmental Origins of a Neurodegenerative Disorder." *Reproductive Toxicology* 23(3):457–470.

46. Savory, J., et al., August 1, 1996. "Can the Controversy of the Role of Aluminum in Alzheimer's Disease Be Resolved? What Are the Suggested Approaches to This Controversy and Methodological Issues to Be Considered?" *Journal of Toxicology and Environmental Health,* Part A, 48(6).

47. Sapolsky, R. *Why Zebras Don't Get Ulcers: An Updated Guide to Stress, Stress-Related Disease and Coping.* New York: W. H. Freeman, 1998.

48. Rizzolatti, G., Craighero, L. 2004. "The Mirror Neuron System." *Annual Review of Neuroscience* 27(27):169–92.

49. Katzman, R., et al. 1988. "Clinical, Pathological, and Neurochemical Changes in Dementia: A Subgroup with Preserved Mental Status and Numerous Neocortical Plaques." *Annals of Neurology* 23(2):138–44.

50. Smith, A. D., Zigmond, M. J. 2003. "Can the Brain Be Protected Through Exercise? Lessons from an Animal Model of Parkinsonism." *Experimental Neurology* 184(1):274–84.

51. Zhang, M., et al. 1990. "The Prevalence of Dementia and Alzheimer's Disease in Shanghai, China: Impact of Age, Gender, and Education." *Annals of Neurology* 27(4):428–37.

52. Whalley, L. J., et al. 2000. "Childhood Mental Ability and Dementia." *Neurology* 55:1455–59.

53. Fritsche, T., et al. 2005. "Associations Between Dementia/Mild Cognitive Impairment and Cognitive Performance and Activity Levels in Youth." *Journal of the American Geriatrics Society* 53(7):1191–96.

54. Snowdon, D. A., et al. 1996. "Linguistic Ability in Early Life and Cognitive Function and Alzheimer's Disease in Late Life. Findings from the Nun Study." *JAMA* 275(903):528–32.

55. Kraemer, G. W. 1998. "Brain Development, Attachment and Impact on Psychic Vulnerability." *Psychiatric Times* 15(5):1–5.

56. Greenough, W. T., Black, J. E., Wallace, C. S. 1987. "Experience and Brain Development." *Child Development* 58(3):539–59.

57. Fritsche et al., op. cit., pp. 1191–96.

58. House, J. S., Robbins, C., Metzner, H. L. 1982. "The Association of Social Relationships and Activities with Mortality: Prospective Evidence from the Tecumseh Community Health Study." *American Journal of Epidemiology* 116(1):123–40.

59. Fabrigoule, C., et al. 1995. "Social and Leisure Activities and Risk of Dementia: A Prospective Longitudinal Study." *Journal of the American Geriatrics Society* 43(5):485–90.

60. Lindstrom, H. A., et al. 2005. "The Relationships Between Television Viewing in Midlife and the Development of Alzheimer's Disease in a Case-Controlled Study." *Brain and Cognition* 58:157–65.

61. Nalsh, J. October 21, 2006. "Chief of the Screen Police: Susan Greenfield Tells John Nalsh Why Our Onscreen Computer Culture Could Create a Dumb Generation." *The Times* (London), p. 2.

62. Rowe, J. W., Kahn, R. L. 1998. "Successful Aging." *Aging (Milano)* 10(2):142–44. Rowe, J. W., Kahn, R. L. July 10, 1987. "Human Aging: Usual and Successful." *Science* 237(4811):143–49. Stuck, A. E., et al. 1999. "Risk Factors for Functional Status Decline in Community-Living Elderly People: A Systematic Literature Review." *Social Science and Medicine* 48(4):445–69.

63. Welin, L., et al. 1992. "Social Network and Activities in Relation to Mortality from Cardiovascular Diseases, Cancer and Other Causes—a 12 Year Follow Up of the Study of Men Born in 1913 and 1923." *Journal of Epidemiology and Community Health* 46(2):127–32. Brown, G. W., Harris, T. *Social Origins of Depression*. London: Tavistock, 1978. Unger, J. B., Johnson, C. A., Marks, G. 1997. "Functional Decline in the Elderly: Evidence for Direct and Stress-Buffering Protective Effects of Social Interactions and Physical Activity." *Annals of Behavioral Medicine* 19(2):152–60.

64. Marmot, M. G., et al. 1975. "Epidemiological Studies of Coronary Heart Disease and Stroke in Japanese Men Living in Japan, Hawaii, and California: Prevalence of

Coronary and Hypertensive Heart Disease and Associated Risk Factors." *American Journal of Epidemiology* 102(6):514–25. Marmot, M. G., Syme, S. L. 1976. "Acculturation and Coronary Heart Disease in Japanese Americans." *American Journal of Epidemiology* 104(6):225–47.

65. House, Robbins, and Metzner, op. cit., pp. 123–40.

66. Berkman, L. F., Breslow, L. *Health and Ways of Living: The Alameda County Study*. New York: Oxford University Press, 1983, pp. 83–85. Moen, P., Dempster-McClain, D., Williams Jr., R. August 1989. "Social Integration and Longevity: An Event History Analysis of Women's Roles and Resilience." *American Sociological Review* 54(4):635–47.

67. Blazer, D. G. 2003. "Depression in Late Life: Review and Commentary." *The Journals of Gerontology Series A: Biological Sciences and Medical Sciences* 58(3):M249–65.

68. Steffens D., et al. 2002. "Hippocampal Volume and Incident Dementia in Geriatric Depression." *American Journal of Geriatric Psychiatry* 10:62–71.

69. Scheidt, R., Humpherys, D., Yorgason, J. September 1999. "Successful Aging: What's Not to Like?" *Journal of Applied Gerontology* 18(3):272–82.

70. Baltes, P. 1993. "The Aging Mind." *Gerontologist* 33(5):580–94.

71. Ibid.

72. www.aarp.org (accessed December 16, 2006).

73. Shore, R. *Rethinking the Brain*. New York: Families and Work Institute, 1997.

74. Finch, C. E., Crimmins, E. M. September 2004. "Inflammatory Exposure and Historical Changes in Human Life-Spans." *Science* 305(8691):17.

75. Golden, M. H. 1998. "Oedematous Malnutrition." *British Medical Bulletin* 54(2):433–44.

Epilogue: Thinking Like a Mountain: The Future of Aging

1. From text of commencement address by Steve Jobs, CEO of Apple Computer and of Pixar Animation Studios, delivered on June 12, 2005.

2. Originally contained in United States public utility law, the "public interest, convenience, and necessity" provision was incorporated into the Radio Act of 1927 to become the operational standard for broadcast licensees.

INDEX

Abramson, John, 147
acetylcholine, 53, 123, 242
    drug side effects and, 118
    ginseng's influence on, 140
    memory and learning capabilities and, 52, 57, 116–17, 122
activities, social. *See also* exercise
    AD prevention/maintenance via, 11, 13, 30, 126, 127, 249–58, 262
    advantageous types of, 249–50
    benefits of, 252–56
    boundaries in, 255
    solitary v. community-based, 250–55
    workplace, 256–58, 262
acupuncture, 138–39
AD. *See* Alzheimer's disease
ADEAR. *See* Alzheimer's Disease Education and Referral Center
Adkins, Janet, 217–18
advance directives, 272
advocacy organizations, AD
    exaggeration/deception by, 5–6, 101–4, 114
    language framing within, 107, 108
    motivations of, 101–2, 114
advocacy/activism, 281. *See also* community-based initiative(s)
    on education, 249, 262
    on elder care, 276–78
    on global warming, 259–60, 263
    on infectious diseases, 258–59, 263
After Virtue (MacIntyre), 42
Ageing Cell, 276
aging. *See* brain aging; successful aging
Albom, Mitch, 252
Alive with Alzheimer's (Greenblatt), 271
alternative medicine. *See* complementary and alternative medicine

aluminum exposure, 242–43
Alzheimer, Alois, x, 57, 78–79
    AD label ambivalence by, 16, 86–87, 95–96, 100
    Auguste D. research by, 80–86, 182–83
    bath treatments by, 87
    death of, 89–90
    Freud's theories v., 88–89
    Pick's theories v., 87–88
Alzheimer's: A Love Story (Davidson), 29
Alzheimer's Association, 91, 115, 255, 288
    AD politics and, 96–97
    brain-aging assessment and, 178, 179, 182
    funding for, 47, 103–4, 114
    locating chapters of, 196
    mission statement of, 101
    services provided by, 195–96, 216, 250
Alzheimer's disease (AD). *See also* brain aging; dementia; diagnosis, AD; myths, AD; science, AD; treatment, AD
    beneficiaries related to, 103–5
    brain aging v., x, 38–39, 56, 91–109, 190
    celebrity associations to, 99–100
    characteristics of 57, 58
    childhood's relation to, 258–60
    coping with changes from, 214–15
    cost, economic, of, 34
    diabetes' association with, 74
    diagnostic terminology concerns and, 32–34, 38–39, 40, 41–45, 46–49
    funding/spending for research of, 98, 100, 105, 113
    genetics in relation to, 8, 62–66, 149–50, 151–59, 172, 221
    institutionalization of, 94–96

ABOUT THE AUTHORS

Peter Whitehouse, M.D., Ph.D. (Psychology), and M.A. (Bioethics), trained at Brown and Johns Hopkins universities. He is currently a professor at Case Western Reserve University. He is a geriatric neurologist, cognitive neuroscientist, and "global" bioethicist. His pioneering, internationally recognized work led to an understanding of how the brain is affected by what he used to call Alzheimer's disease and to the development of current drugs for the condition. His integrative clinical practice is built around the power of stories to assist those with aging-associated cognitive challenges. He is a founder with his wife of the Intergenerational School, an innovative, successful urban public school in Cleveland.

Daniel George, M.Sc., is pursuing a Ph.D. in medical anthropology at Oxford University in England. Also an aspiring artist, he is from Cleveland, Ohio, and earned his B.A. from the College of Wooster in Ohio and his M.Sc. from Oxford. He has been a research assistant to Dr. Whitehouse since 2004.